Childhood Development and Behavior

Editors

KATHLEEN G. DAVIS
CHET D. JOHNSON

D0914493

PEDIATRIC CLINICS OF NORTH AMERICA

www.pediatric.theclinics.com

Consulting Editor
BONITA F. STANTON

October 2016 • Volume 63 • Number 5

ELSEVIER

1600 John F. Kennedy Boulevard ● Suite 1800 ● Philadelphia, Pennsylvania, 19103-2899

http://www.theclinics.com

THE PEDIATRIC CLINICS OF NORTH AMERICA Volume 63, Number 5
October 2016 ISSN 0031-3955, ISBN-13: 978-0-323-46325-6

Editor: Kerry Holland
Developmental Editor: Casey Jackson

The Pediatric Clinics of North America (ISSN 0031-3955) is published bimonthly by Elsevier Inc., 360 Park Avenue South, New York, NY 10010-1710. Months of issue are February, April, June, August, October, and December. Periodicals postage paid at New York, NY and additional mailing offices. Subscription prices are $200.00 per year (US individuals), $556.00 per year (US institutions), $270.00 per year (Canadian individuals), $740.00 per year (Canadian institutions), $325.00 per year (international individuals), $740.00 per year (international institutions), $100.00 per year (US students and residents), and $165.00 per year (international and Canadian residents and students). To receive students/resident rare, orders must be accompanied by name of affiliated institution, date of term, and the signature of program/residency coordinator on institution letterhead. Orders will be billed at individual rate until proof of status is received. Foreign air speed delivery is included in all *Clinics* subscription prices. All prices are subject to change without notice. **POSTMASTER:** Send address changes to *The Pediatric Clinics of North America*, Elsevier Health Sciences Division, Subscription Customer Service, 3251 Riverport Lane, Maryland Heights, MO 63043. **Customer Service: 1-800-654-2452 (US and Canada). From outside of the US and Canada: 1-314-447-8871. Fax: 1-314-447-8029. For print support, E-mail: JournalsCustomerService-usa@elsevier.com. For online support, E-mail: JournalsOnlineSupport-usa@elsevier.com.**

Reprints. For copies of 100 or more, of articles in this publication, please contact the Commercial Reprints Department, Elsevier Inc., 360 Park Avenue South, New York, NY 10010-1710. Tel.: 212-633-3074; Fax: 212-633-3820; E-mail: reprints@elsevier.com.

The Pediatric Clinics of North America is also published in Spanish by McGraw-Hill Inter-americana Editores S.A., Mexico City, Mexico; in Portuguese by Riechmann and Affonso Editores, Rua Comandante Coelho 1085, CEP 21250, Rio de Janeiro, Brazil; and in Greek by Althayia SA, Athens, Greece.

The Pediatric Clinics of North America is covered in *MEDLINE/PubMed (Index Medicus), Excerpta Medica, Current Contents, Current Contents/Clinical Medicine, Science Citation Index, ASCA, ISI/BIOMED*, and *BIOSIS*.

Printed in the United States of America.

PROGRAM OBJECTIVE
The goal of the *Pediatric Clinics of North America* is to keep practicing physicians and residents up to date with current clinical practice in pediatrics by providing timely articles reviewing the state-of-the-art in patient care.

TARGET AUDIENCE
All practicing pediatricians, physicians and healthcare professionals who provide patient care to pediatric patients.

LEARNING OBJECTIVES
Upon completion of this activity, participants will be able to:
1. Review the effects of factors such as military deployment, gun violence, and increased screen time on children's developmental health.
2. Discuss the identification and management of autism and antisocial behaviour in children.
3. Recognize developments in pediatric telemental health, behavioral therapies, and palliative care.

ACCREDITATION
The Elsevier Office of Continuing Medical Education (EOCME) is accredited by the Accreditation Council for Continuing Medical Education (ACCME) to provide continuing medical education for physicians.

The EOCME designates this enduring material for a maximum of 15 *AMA PRA Category 1 Credit*(s)™. Physicians should claim only the credit commensurate with the extent of their participation in the activity.

All other health care professionals requesting continuing education credit for this enduring material will be issued a certificate of participation.

DISCLOSURE OF CONFLICTS OF INTEREST
The EOCME assesses conflict of interest with its instructors, faculty, planners, and other individuals who are in a position to control the content of CME activities. All relevant conflicts of interest that are identified are thoroughly vetted by EOCME for fair balance, scientific objectivity, and patient care recommendations. EOCME is committed to providing its learners with CME activities that promote improvements or quality in healthcare and not a specific proprietary business or a commercial interest.

The planning committee, staff, authors and editors listed below have identified no financial relationships or relationships to products or devices they or their spouse/life partner have with commercial interest related to the content of this CME activity:
Patricia G. Alvarez, MD; Matthew J. Baker, DO; Dimitri A. Christakis, MD, MPH; John D. Cowden, MD, MPH; Kathleen G. Davis, PhD, MSEd; Anjali Fortna; Jessica Foster, MD, MPH; Paul J. Frick, PhD; Eliza Gordon-Lipkin, MD; Kerry Holland; Chet D. Johnson, MD, FAAP; Kelly Kreisler, MD, MPH; Indu Kumari; Peter J. Mogayzel, MD, PhD, MBA; Suzie C. Nelson, MD; Eve-Lynn Nelson, PhD; Gwenn Schurgin O'Keeffe, MD; Georgina Peacock, MD, MPH; Jenny S. Radesky, MD; Judy Schaechter, MD, MBA; Susan Sharp, DO; Timothy Ryan Smith, MD; Bonita F. Stanton, MD; Megan Suermann; Susan G. Timmer, PhD; Anthony J. Urquiza, PhD; Natalie E. West, MD, MHS; Christina G. Weston, MD.

UNAPPROVED/OFF-LABEL USE DISCLOSURE
The EOCME requires CME faculty to disclose to the participants:
1. When products or procedures being discussed are off-label, unlabelled, experimental, and/or investigational (not US Food and Drug Administration [FDA] approved); and
2. Any limitations on the information presented, such as data that are preliminary or that represent ongoing research, interim analyses, and/or unsupported opinions. Faculty may discuss information about pharmaceutical agents that is outside of FDA-approved labelling. This information is intended solely for CME and is not intended to promote off-label use of these medications. If you have any questions, contact the medical affairs department of the manufacturer for the most recent prescribing information.

TO ENROLL
To enroll in the *Pediatric Clinics of North America* Continuing Medical Education program, call customer service at 1-800-654-2452 or sign up online at http://www.theclinics.com/home/cme. The CME program is available to subscribers for an additional annual fee of USD 290.

METHOD OF PARTICIPATION

In order to claim credit, participants must complete the following:

1. Complete enrolment as indicated above.
2. Read the activity.
3. Complete the CME Test and Evaluation. Participants must achieve a score of 70% on the test. All CME Tests and Evaluations must be completed online.

CME INQUIRIES/SPECIAL NEEDS

For all CME inquiries or special needs, please contact elsevierCME@elsevier.com.

Contributors

CONSULTING EDITOR

BONITA F. STANTON, MD
Founding Dean, School of Medicine, Professor of Pediatrics, Seton Hall University, South Orange, New Jersey

EDITORS

KATHLEEN G. DAVIS, PhD, MSEd
Associate Professor of Pediatrics, Director of Pediatric Palliative Care and Ethics, Department of Pediatrics, University of Kansas Medical Center, Kansas City, Kansas

CHET D. JOHNSON, MD, FAAP
Olathe Health System, Vice President, Senior Medical and Operations Officer, Olathe Medical Services, Olathe, Kansas

AUTHORS

PATRICIA G. ALVAREZ, MD
Department of Pediatrics, University of Miami Miller School of Medicine and Holtz Children's Hospital at Jackson Health Systems, Miami, Florida

MATTHEW J. BAKER, DO
Assistant Professor, Psychiatry, Wright State University Boonshoft School of Medicine, Dayton, Ohio; Staff Psychiatrist, Wright-Patterson Medical Center, Wright-Patterson Air Force Base, Ohio

DIMITRI A. CHRISTAKIS, MD, MPH
Professor of Pediatrics; Director, Center for Child Health, Behavior and Development, Seattle Children's Hospital, Seattle, Washington

JOHN D. COWDEN, MD, MPH
Associate Professor, Department of Pediatrics, Medical Director of Equity and Diversity, Children's Mercy Kansas City, University of Missouri-Kansas City, Kansas City, Missouri

KATHLEEN G. DAVIS, PhD, MSEd
Associate Professor of Pediatrics, Director of Pediatric Palliative Care and Ethics, Department of Pediatrics, University of Kansas Medical Center, Kansas City, Kansas

JESSICA FOSTER, MD, MPH
Chief, Section of Developmental Pediatrics, Akron Children's Hospital, Akron, Ohio

PAUL J. FRICK, PhD
Professor, Department of Psychology Louisiana State University, Baton Rouge, Louisiana; Professor, Learning Sciences Institute of Australia, Australian Catholic University, Melbourne, Victoria, Australia

ELIZA GORDON-LIPKIN, MD
Fellow, Department of Neurology and Developmental Medicine, Kennedy Krieger Institute, Baltimore, Maryland

KELLY KREISLER, MD, MPH
Assistant Professor, Department of Pediatrics, University of Kansas School of Medicine, Program Director for Community Health Improvement and Outreach Initiatives, University of Kansas Hospital, Kansas City, Kansas

PETER J. MOGAYZEL Jr, MD, PhD, MBA
Professor of Pediatrics; Director, Cystic Fibrosis Center, Johns Hopkins Cystic Fibrosis Center, Baltimore, Maryland

EVE-LYNN NELSON, PhD
Professor, KU Pediatrics; Director, KU Center for Telemedicine & Telehealth; University of Kansas Medical Center; Fairway, Kansas

SUZIE C. NELSON, MD
Assistant Professor, Psychiatry, Wright State University Boonshoft School of Medicine, Dayton, Ohio; Director, Child Psychiatry Services, Wright-Patterson Medical Center, Wright-Patterson Air Force Base, Ohio

GWENN SCHURGIN O'KEEFFE, MD
CEO and Chief Editor, Pediatrics Now, Wayland, Massachusetts

GEORGINA PEACOCK, MD, MPH
Director, Division of Human Development and Disability, National Center on Birth Defects and Developmental Disabilities, Centers for Disease Control and Prevention, Atlanta, Georgia

JENNY S. RADESKY, MD
Assistant Professor of Developmental Behavioral Pediatrics, University of Michigan Medical School, University of Michigan, Ann Arbor, Michigan

JUDY SCHAECHTER, MD, MBA
Department of Pediatrics, University of Miami Miller School of Medicine and Holtz Children's Hospital at Jackson Health Systems, Miami, Florida

SUSAN SHARP, DO
Assistant Professor, Division of Child Psychiatry, Psychiatry Department, University of Kansas Medical Center, Kansas City, Kansas

TIMOTHY RYAN SMITH, MD
Assistant Professor of Pediatrics, University of Kansas Medical Center, Kansas City, Kansas

SUSAN G. TIMMER, PhD
Associate Professor, Director of Mental Health Research, CAARE Diagnostic and Treatment Center, UC Davis Children's Hospital, Sacramento, California

ANTHONY J. URQUIZA, PhD
Professor, Executive Director, CAARE Diagnostic and Treatment Center, UC Davis Children's Hospital, Sacramento, California

NATALIE E. WEST, MD, MHS
Assistant Professor of Medicine; Division of Pulmonary and Critical Care Medicine, Johns Hopkins University, Baltimore, Maryland

CHRISTINA G. WESTON, MD
Associate Professor, Psychiatry, Director, Child and Adolescent Fellowship Training, Wright State University Boonshoft School of Medicine, Dayton, Ohio

Contents

Children of immigrant families experience developmental processes in the contexts of migration and settlement, presenting immigration-specific challenges. Child health providers can use awareness of the cultural-ecological model of immigrant child development to explore how acculturation, ethnic identity formation, and bilingualism affect the children and families under their care. Cross-cultural strategies for evaluating and supporting immigrant child development are presented to guide the provider in clinical interactions and community efforts.

Many US military families have faced separations of at least one family member for extended periods of time. This article shows how changes in military culture have increased the repercussions for military families, and especially for military-connected children. This article provides an introduction to aspects of military culture that are most applicable to children, an overview of important aspects of childhood development, a discussion of the impact of deployment on the emotional development and behavior of children left at home and their caregivers, and a review of some interventions and resources available to help these families navigate these challenges.

Firearm injury is a leading cause of death and injury for children and adolescents, able to cause disability and interfere with normal development. Child developmental stages, variance of behavior, and mental health may all put children at risk for firearm injury or lead to increased morbidity after experiencing firearm violence. Family, community, and contextual factors can accentuate the risk of violence. Adults and social structures have the responsibility to protect children and adolescents from firearm violence.

This article describes common mental health problems in children and adolescents, and the types of specialized, evidence-based treatments that are most effective in treating these needs. The value of using an evidence-based treatment is now widely acknowledged, and the number of interventions with empirical support is increasing. This article provides an overview of the effects of trauma on developing children, with an emphasis on common maladaptive responses in infancy, toddlerhood, young childhood, middle childhood, and adolescence. This is followed by descriptions of several well-researched interventions that have the greatest utility for each distinct phase of child development.

Numerous individuals with chronic disease age into adulthood each year, necessitating transition from a pediatric to an adult medical care team. Transition should start early in adolescence and occur gradually over years, preparing the individual for the transfer to the adult team. Cystic fibrosis (CF) has a growing population of adults, as survival over the past several decades has increased. The CF Foundation has implemented guidelines for the transition process. The transition process for individuals with CF provides an example that could be adapted into other chronic disease populations, to provide a successful and meaningful transition into adult care.

Children and adolescents with complex chronic conditions often receive pediatric palliative care (PPC) from health care professionals. However, children's needs exist both in a health care context and in the community where children interact with peers, including school, places of worship, sports, activities, and organizations. Partnerships between PPC professionals in health care settings and teachers, coaches, spiritual leaders, activity directors, and others, may lead to greater health and well-being. Children near the end of life or those with out-of-hospital do-not-resuscitate orders may also find palliation in their community. Cooperation between all caregivers benefit the child and family.

Because of the widening gap between need for child mental health services and availability of child specialists, secure videoconferencing options are more needed than ever to address access challenges across underserved settings. This article reviews real-time videoconferencing evidence across telemental health with children and adolescents. It summarizes emerging guidelines that inform best practices for child telemental

health using videoconferencing. It presents a case example of best practices across behavioral health specialties. Videoconferencing is an effective approach to improving access to behavioral health interventions for
children and adolescents. Telemental health shows promise for disseminating evidence-based treatments to underserved communities.

Timothy Ryan Smith

Effective well-child care includes developmental surveillance and
screening to identify developmental delays and subsequent interventions.
Electronic health records (EHRs) have been widely adopted to improve efficiency and appropriate clinical practice. Developmental surveillance
tools have been introduced. This article summarizes a conceptual framework for application and highlights the principles and tools of EHRs
applied to developmental assessment, including interoperability, health information exchange, clinical decision support systems, consumer health
informatics, dashboards, and patient portals. Further investigation and
dedicated resources will be required for successful application to developmental surveillance and screening.

PEDIATRIC CLINICS OF NORTH AMERICA

Foreword

Insights and Influences on Our Children's Development and Behaviors

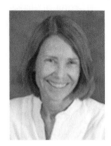

Bonita F. Stanton, MD
Consulting Editor

Our understanding of behavior and child development continues to advance through further study and progress in assessment tools and techniques. At the same time, greater expansion in travel and migration and rapid changes in the manner in which children interact with technology doubtless impact actual behavior and development. Who among us has not experienced widely divergent emotions regarding the array of experiences and exposures confronting children in the twenty-first century and their possible impacts on the cognitive and/or emotional growth?

This thoughtfully written issue examines children growing up in immigrant families and in families in which one or both parents are deployed in the military. It addresses the issue of gun violence, the ever-increasing screen time, and the impact of social media on behavior and development. It examines technological advances in screening and the prospects for and implications of early diagnosis on outcomes for autism and antisocial behavior. Through the lens of cystic fibrosis, it examines the developmental and behavioral implications of increased life expectancy among children with formerly fatal diseases as they exit childhood and enter what now holds the potential for a long adulthood. The issue concludes with two articles addressing advances in our understanding of therapies for children with special needs and an expanded community presence of palliative care, including its presence in the school system.

As pediatricians and other child specialists read this issue of *Pediatric Clinics of North America*, they likely will be struck with the realization that many of the exciting advances in technology and experiences that allow us to better understand child behavior and development in our communities and across the globe are the same advances that are influencing the behavioral and developmental arcs of today's children

Pediatr Clin N Am 63 (2016) xv–xvi
http://dx.doi.org/10.1016/j.pcl.2016.06.017
0031-3955/16/$ – see front matter © 2016 Published by Elsevier Inc.

pediatric.theclinics.com

and youth. At this point, this observation is not a value statement but rather an aware-ness with a sense that further analysis is warranted.

Bonita F. Stanton, MD
School of Medicine
Seton Hall University
400 South Orange Avenue
South Orange, NJ 07079, USA

E-mail address:
bonita.stanton@shu.edu

Preface

Contemporary Pediatric Public Health Challenges

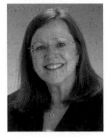 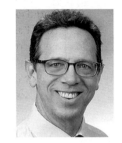

Kathleen G. Davis, PhD, MSEd   Chet D. Johnson, MD, FAAP
Editors

The pediatrician who cared for children from the neighborhood or, at the very least, the community no longer exists in many places. Today, pediatricians are more likely to care for children and families from all walks of life. Some may still be children we know from our neighborhoods. Many more, however, are likely to be children from other lands and various cultures. We may speak the same language as some of your patients and their parents and need a translator to enable us to have a meaningful connection with others. Some conditions and social issues look the same as they did a generation ago, but our patients and their families present with other needs that look dramatically different than those that children used to encounter. Children come to us with different social and emotional concerns, and as we care about and care for their physical and mental health, our concern also extends to their families. And we care about how children are doing in all environments: at home, at school, and in their communities.

In this era, children and their families are impacted by social and political changes in our homes (social media and screen time), in our communities (refugee populations), in our health care networks (EMR in every tertiary pediatric center), and in our larger world (multiple military deployments of fathers and mothers). Our young patients are involved in a variety of activities at school, at places of worship, and in the community. When a child is diagnosed with a life-threatening condition or when there is an act of gun violence that affects one child, that child's entire community is touched.

In addition to helping children and families by treating a child's physical or mental illness, pediatricians today are called upon to guide children and their parents through what sometimes seems like a mine field with potential danger looming with the next step. Although our responsibilities may seem daunting at times—and especially difficult to address in the 15-minute appointment—there are new ways to help children and families and expertise that is developing around us. As we make the adjustments to incorporate some of the "newness" that the twenty-first century has presented to us,

Pediatr Clin N Am 63 (2016) xvii–xviii
http://dx.doi.org/10.1016/j.pcl.2016.06.016
0031-3955/16/$ – see front matter © 2016 Published by Elsevier Inc.

pediatric.theclinics.com

we may find that, in many ways, our role is not more difficult; it is just richer and more robust.

This issue explores the impact of contemporary public health challenges for pediatric care, promising models for caring for chronically ill children, and state-of-the-art therapies for complex childhood conditions. It is our hope that that issue of *Pediatric Clinics of North America* will provide you with some new solutions to old problems; some new solutions to new problems; and a great deal of "food for thought" as you ponder not only how your practice looks today but also how it will appear in the future. Thank you for your interest.

Kathleen G. Davis, PhD, MSEd
University of Kansas Health System
Pediatric Palliative Care and Ethics
KUMC
3901 Rainbow Boulevard–MS4004
Kansas City, KS 66160, USA

Chet D. Johnson, MD, FAAP
Olathe Health System
Olathe Medical Services
13045 South Mur-Len Road
Olathe, KS 66062, USA

E-mail addresses:
kdavis2@kumc.edu (K.G. Davis)
chet.johnson@olathehealth.org (C.D. Johnson)

Development in Children of Immigrant Families

John D. Cowden, MD, MPH[a],*, Kelly Kreisler, MD, MPH[b]

KEYWORDS

- Immigrant • Refugee • Children • Pediatric • Development

KEY POINTS

- Understanding contexts of migration and settlement is an essential component in the developmental and behavioral evaluation of an immigrant child.
- Acculturation, ethnic identity formation, and bilingualism are fundamental developmental processes for the immigrant child.
- Although bilingualism brings multiple cognitive and social benefits, dual-language learners are at increased risk of low academic achievement.
- Risks of stereotyping and unconscious bias are high in cross-cultural interactions; understanding the unique experience of each immigrant child relies on applying general knowledge to the specific interaction from a stance of cultural humility.

INTRODUCTION

Immigration is one of the major societal issues of the day, bringing challenge and opportunity to those working to support the health and well-being of children. In the United States, the youngest segment of society has diversified fastest, with children from immigrant families increasing from 15% to 24% of the younger than age 18 population between 1994 and 2014.[1] By 2050, they are expected to make up one-third of all US children (**Fig. 1**).[2] Parents of immigrant children in the United States come from all regions of the world and show diverse settlement patterns (**Fig. 2**), whereas refugee families tend to come from specific regions in the Middle East, Africa, and Asia. Just less than two-thirds of refugees who resettled in the United States in 2014 came from Iraq, Burma, and Somalia.[3]

In pediatric settings, as the number of children from immigrant families increases, the need to understand the special issues they face becomes more pressing. Recent

The authors have nothing to disclose.
[a] Department of Pediatrics, Children's Mercy Kansas City, University of Missouri-Kansas City, 2401 Gillham Road, Kansas City, MO 64108, USA; [b] Department of Pediatrics, University of Kansas School of Medicine, University of Kansas Hospital, The University of Kansas Physicians Medical Office Building, 3901 Rainbow Boulevard, MS 4004, Kansas City, KS 66160, USA
* Corresponding author.
E-mail address: jdcowden@cmh.edu

Pediatr Clin N Am 63 (2016) 775–793
http://dx.doi.org/10.1016/j.pcl.2016.06.005
0031-3955/16/$ – see front matter © 2016 Elsevier Inc. All rights reserved.

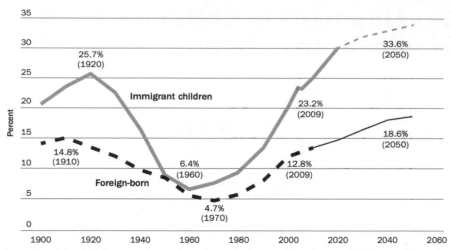

Fig. 1. Total foreign-born as share of total population and immigrant children as share of all children, 1900 to 2050. (Population estimates for 1900–1950 are based on Integrated Public-Use Microdata Series; Edmonston B, Passel JS. Ethnic demography: U.S. immigration and ethnic variations. In: Edmonston B, Passel JS, editors. Immigration and ethnicity: the integration of America's newest arrivals. Washington: Urban Institute Press; 1994; Data for 1960–2000 and 2010–2050 are from Passel JS, Cohn D. U.S. population projections: 2005–2010. Washington: Pew Hispanic Center; 2008; and Data for 2001–2009 are from tabulations of the March Current Population Survey with imputations for legal status and corrections for undercoverage. See technical appendix; and *From* Passel JS. Demography of immigrant youth: past, present, and future. Future Child 2011;21(1):23; with permission.)

publications, such as the *Immigrant Child Health Toolkit* from the American Academy of Pediatrics (AAP)[4] and the article by Linton and colleagues,[5] address the broad health needs of children of immigrant families. Here we focus on what is known about the effects of immigration on child development. Understanding of this area has expanded rapidly through work in multiple disciplines, including psychology, sociology, psychiatry, public health, public policy, and developmental pediatrics.

This article offers the practicing pediatric provider an orientation to current knowledge about child development in the immigrant context and a clinical approach to caring for immigrant children. In it, we provide a description of how child development theories have incorporated immigration, followed by a discussion of issues with special relevance to children living in an immigrant context. Finally, we outline tools and interventions applicable in the clinical setting.

Variations of "child of an immigrant family" are used throughout this article, as the phrase captures two distinct situations of interest to the pediatric practitioner: a child who immigrates from one country to another, also called first generation; and a child who is born in a new country to which a family has immigrated, or second generation. For brevity, the term "immigrant child" is also used to denote a child of an immigrant family, regardless of generational status. Although developmental processes and outcomes can differ widely for first- and second-generation immigrant children, research in this area is not yet well-developed, so generally they are treated together here (except where noted). Specific types of immigrant children, including refugees, asylum-seekers, stateless persons, unaccompanied immigrant children, and undocumented immigrants, are defined in **Box 1**.

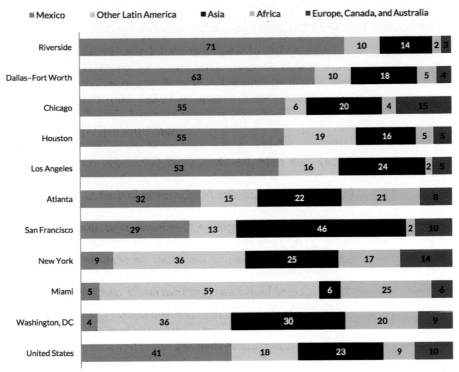

■ Mexico   ■ Other Latin America   ■ Asia   ■ Africa   ■ Europe, Canada, and Australia

Riverside	71	10	14	2 3
Dallas–Fort Worth	63	10	18	5 4
Chicago	55	6	20	4 15
Houston	55	19	16	5 5
Los Angeles	53	16	24	2 5
Atlanta	32	15	22	21	8
San Francisco	29	13	46	2 10
New York	9	36	25	17	14
Miami	5	59	6	25	6
Washington, DC	4	36	30	20	9
United States	41	18	23	9	10

Fig. 2. Children of immigrants from birth to age 17 by parents' region of origin, 2013. This figure only presents the data for the United States overall and the 10 metropolitan areas with the highest population of children of immigrants. (Urban Institute tabulations from the Integrated Public Use Microdata Series datasets drawn from the 2012 and 2013 American Community Surveys; and *From* Woods T, Hanson D, Saxton S, et al. Children of immigrants: 2013 state trends update. Washington, DC: The Urban Institute; 2016, with permission.)

Box 1
Terms related to immigrant children

Term	Definition
Child of an immigrant family	A child who has at least one foreign-born parent
First-generation immigrant child	A child born outside the country to which they immigrated
Second-generation immigrant child	A child born in the settlement country to a foreign-born parent
Refugee/asylum-seeker[a]	Someone who has been forced to flee his or her country because of persecution, war, or violence and has or seeks legal residence in another country[b]
Stateless person	Someone who is not considered as a national by any country[b]
Unaccompanied immigrant child	A child who immigrates without a parent or adult guardian
Unauthorized immigrant	A foreign-born resident without legal status (eg, temporary worker, lawful permanent resident, citizen)

[a] By definition, refugees have received legal status, whereas asylum seekers are requesting it based on perceived persecution or danger in their home country.
[b] For details of refugee, asylum-seeker, and stateless person demographics and procedures, see United Nations High Commissioner for Refugees (UNHCR) Web site: www.unhcr.org and US State Department Refugee Admissions Web site: http://www.state.gov/j/prm/ra/index.htm.

INCORPORATING IMMIGRATION INTO CHILD DEVELOPMENT THEORY

Early theories of child development focused on defining the processes a child goes through between infancy and adolescence: the physical, cognitive, psychosocial, and moral changes experienced in a common, expected progression. In recent decades, the role of a child's environment has become a more prominent part of developmental modeling, especially since the emergence of the ecological model of human development, first described in 1979 by Bronfenbrenner.[6] The ecological model, based on the interactions between an individual and the multiple environments around them, offers important perspectives on how the processes of development are affected by the contexts in which children live.

The ecological model describes four nested levels of the environment (microsystem, mesosystem, exosystem, and macrosystem) that impact a child's development at all ages (**Fig. 3**). The microsystems are the most immediate contexts of a child's life (family, school, peer relations, religious setting) in which they are affected by direct interactions with others. The mesosystem is formed by interactions between

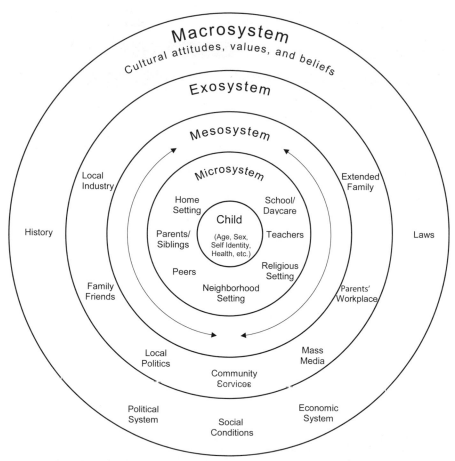

Fig. 3. Ecological model of human development. (*Data from* Bronfenbrenner U. The ecology of human development: experiments by nature and design. Cambridge (MA): Harvard University Press; 1979.)

microsystems (eg, parents interacting with teachers or monitoring a child's peer inter-actions). The exosystem includes elements, such as extended family, neighborhoods, parents' workplaces, local policies, mass media, and industry, which indirectly affect children through interactions with microsystems.The macrosystem is the overarching cultural setting that a child experiences through its influence on the other contexts. It includes cultural beliefs and ideologies; societal structure; and social, political, and economic conditions, among other things.

For a child growing up in a stable setting, these systems create a complex set of in-fluences that play a formative role in development. When children emigrate from one country to another, the complexity increases considerably. Some microsystems fall away and are replaced by new ones, resulting in mesosytem shifts and fractures. Exo-systems and macrosystems collide, opening questions of identity, belonging, and the reconciliation of differing cultural beliefs and norms.

Adaptations to the basic ecological model have been made to account for the way immigration affects the nested systems. In 2007, Perreira and Smith[7] described the cultural-ecological model of migration and development, in which they introduced the migration context and the settlement context, each with specific characteristics that in-fluence ethnic identification, psychosocial outcomes, and general well-being of the immigrant child (**Fig. 4**).[7] The migration context includes migration motives (eg, voluntary vs forced) and migration events (what happens along the way). The settlement context is characterized by acculturation strategies (assimilation, separation, marginalization, or biculturation) and acculturation experiences (how the settlement community's policies, school/work conditions, and attitude toward ethnicity and immigration affect the child).

In this model, migration and settlement contexts are not elements of a microsystem, exosystem, or macrosystem, but represent modifiers of these systems, or lenses through which developmental challenges specific to the immigrant child are identified. For the clinician assessing an immigrant child's progress through the standard devel-opmental processes (physical, cognitive, psychosocial, and so forth), the ecological model and its migration-specific adaptation offer a framework for considering forces at play in an immigrant child's developmental trajectory.

DEVELOPMENTAL CHALLENGES RELATED TO IMMIGRATION

The interplay between universal developmental processes and migrant and settlement contexts results in experiences specific to the children of immigrants. Three

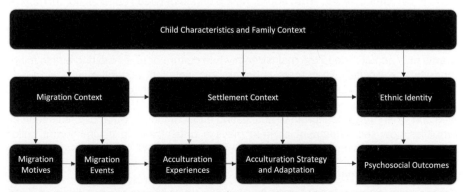

Fig. 4. Cultural-ecological model of migration, acculturation, and ethnic identification. (*Adapted from* Perreira KM, Smith L. A cultural-ecological model of migration and develop-ment: focusing on Latino immigrant youth. Prev Res 2007;14(4):6.)

fundamental immigrant developmental processes are (1) acculturation, (2) ethnic identity formation, and (3) bilingualism.[8]

Acculturation

Acculturation was originally described as a unilateral process by which immigrant communities could assimilate into the dominant receiving culture. Newer theories reject the idea of unilateral acculturation in favor of a bilateral exchange, in which immigrants both affect and are affected by the environment where they settle. Two current acculturation models can help the clinician frame an immigrant child's experience: the four-fold model and the interactive acculturation model.

In the four-fold model, there are four basic strategies available to immigrant families and their children[9]: (1) assimilation (replacement of the original culture with the new); (2) separation (rejection of the new culture while maintaining the original); (3) marginalization (rejection or denial of access to the new culture along with loss of the original, either willingly or by force); and (4) integration (acceptance of the new culture while maintaining the culture of origin).

The interactive acculturation model considers not only the viewpoint of the newcomer (as in the four-fold model), but also the orientation of the host community to the acculturation of immigrants.[10] This model underlies the description of the settlement context in the cultural-ecological approach described previously. The orientation to acculturation among immigrants (Do they wish to retain their culture? Adopt the new culture? Both?) can be compared with the readiness of the host community to accommodate newcomers (Are there policies that are proimmigration or anti-immigration? Are school and work structures set up to receive those from different cultures? What are the pre-existing attitudes about racial/ethnic interactions?), resulting in a dynamic set of possibilities representative of experiences in a multicultural society.

Children and parents in immigrant families often experience acculturation in different ways. As children go to school, they are rapidly socialized (ie, explicitly taught values, norms, and behaviors) and enculturated (ie, implicitly pick up cultural nuances) in the host culture, and are unlikely to "choose" an acculturation strategy the way an adult might. Parents often continue to socialize them at home in the ways of their culture of origin, but lack the same opportunities for either socialization or enculturation in their new environment. These differences in experience can lead to acculturation gaps in the family, with children more strongly tied to the new culture and parents struggling to maintain what they see as an appropriate balance between cultures, for themselves and their children.[11]

In addition to the "how" of acculturation, a clinician also should consider to which host culture a child or family is acculturating. In a multicultural US society, new immigrants may acculturate to the mainstream white culture or to an existing ethnic minority culture, especially when there is geographic isolation, cultural affinity, or a large coethnic community. Discrimination is a common experience for immigrant children, particularly when the receiving culture is negatively oriented to immigration and minorities and when they acculturate to an existing ethnic minority. Such discrimination exemplifies how the settlement context plays a critical role in an immigrant child's developmental trajectory.

Ethnic Identity Formation

For the child of an immigrant family, feeling different and being treated differently in the receiving culture can provide the basis for a sense of ethnic identity.[12] This typically begins in preadolescence and continues throughout the adolescent years, when the confluence of personal identity (Who am I?) and social identity (To what groups do I belong?) leads to an abstract sense of self. By definition, ethnic identity relates to ethnic group belonging, but the labels used to self-categorize are dynamic and multi-layered. Although panethnic categories, such as Latino and Asian, are commonly used in the United States, they usually do not exist in the heritage country immigrants leave behind, creating a potentially confusing situation for immigrant youth. More specific identities, such as Mexican American or Chinese American, and multiethnic combinations (eg, American, black, and Somali or Latino, Argentinian, and white) provide more precise terms for expression of identity, although individuals also move through varied expressions of ethnic identity depending on the context.

Strong ethnic identity generally has been shown to be protective for immigrant adolescents and young adults, particularly against anxiety, depression, conduct problems, and substance abuse.[12] Biculturalism, which can occur when ethnic identity includes both heritage and receiving cultures (eg, Nigerian and US identification), also is associated with enhanced well-being, although details of how it differs among ethnic groups, between first- and second-generation immigrants, and across the age span is not well understood.

A challenge facing many immigrant children is the perpetual foreigner syndrome, which describes the way ethnic minority members can be treated as foreign by the dominant ethnic group in a community, no matter their birthplace or citizenship.[13] When a Japanese, Indian, or Mexican American is asked where they "really" come from, or are complimented on how they speak English without an accent, their sense of identity and belonging can be threatened as they try to reconcile their US identity with the assumptions others make about who they are. Although this can be hurtful, it also can push immigrant youth toward an ethnic identity that becomes central to a strong sense of self.

Bilingualism

As the population of immigrant children grows, so does the need to understand how to support dual-language learners (DLLs), a diverse group of children and youth either learning two languages from the start (simultaneous bilinguals) or a second language on top of a first (sequential bilinguals). Neurocognitive and psycholinguistic research has shown that children can successfully learn two languages simultaneously from birth, naturally laying down separate, but connected language systems.[14,15] The basic stages of DLL language development are similar to monolinguals; however, some important distinctions have been found. Although simultaneous bilinguals may begin speaking later than monolinguals, they are not thought to have language delay. Instead, processes by which DLLs access linguistic information could explain the observations that they can lag in vocabulary and word retrieval, but match or exceed monolinguals in phonologic awareness and word decoding. Given sufficient quality and quantity of exposure, DLLs can reach native level proficiency in both languages. Evidence of cognitive and behavioral advantages also have been found among DLLs, including superior executive function, inhibitory control, task-orientation, instruction-following, and sociolinguistic awareness.[16,17]

Growing research on DLL development has revealed a complex picture that shows the utility of the ecological model in considering children's language development paths. DLLs have a wide variety of language outcomes influenced by individual characteristics; the home, school, and peer settings; the interactions between parents and school; the larger social sphere; and the timing of their exposure to a second language. Such complexity makes it unlikely that a single multilingual learning theory will be able to explain the diversity of outcomes for DLLs. Nevertheless, certain factors seem to be helpful for achieving bilingual proficiency, including individual (younger age, motivation, aptitude), family (value placed on heritage language and bilingualism; higher parental education, literacy, and socioeconomic status), and school (experienced and supportive of DLLs) characteristics.[18] When support for bilingualism is lacking, young children may never develop proficiency in their heritage language. Older children and youth who immigrate with established heritage language proficiency may experience a subtractive process, replacing their heritage language with the new language, rather than the additive process that leads to bilingualism.[18]

As with acculturation and ethnic identity, language gaps can form between members of immigrant families because of differences in language ability and in the value placed on heritage language maintenance. Adolescents might use the ability to speak the dominant cultural language (eg, English) to isolate parents from their activities and might refuse to speak their heritage language as a form of separation from parental authority. Conversely, shared language and cultural value in the family can offer immigrant children and adolescents the benefits of bilingualism, biculturalism, and a strong ethnic identity, and family cohesion.

Common Pitfalls for the Provider

The child development theories and immigration-related processes described above provide only a brief introduction to the challenges faced by immigrant children. A variety of other theories also can be used to understand immigrant children's development and behavior,[19] which is influenced by a wide range of factors not explored here.[19] Two potential pitfalls exist for the provider: not knowing enough about immigrant children's development, and knowing just enough to think in generalizations. Stereotyping, automatic thinking, and unconscious bias put us at risk of treating families from an unfamiliar culture too simplistically.[20] As with all families, the best approach is to ask specific questions without assumption, based on knowledge of the questions that should be asked to those living the dynamic, multicultural reality of immigration. In this way, culturally and linguistically individualized care be given to all children, no matter their families' origins.

CLINICAL APPROACHES TO CHILDREN OF IMMIGRANT FAMILIES
Cross-Cultural Care

Providing high-quality care to immigrant families relies on understanding the role of culture in how families access health care and how clinicians interact with them in the clinical setting. Differences in cultural norms related to eye contact, personal space, communication style, and displays of respect can lead to misunderstandings, which ultimately contribute to disparities in health and health care. Cultural competence and related concepts (eg, cultural respect, humility, awareness) have become a top priority in health care, as reflected by the publication of the Culturally and Linguistically Appropriate Services standards by the US Office of Minority Health.[21] The Culturally and Linguistically Appropriate Services standards offer an excellent reference for providers and health care institutions in their efforts to provide culturally competent care to children of immigrant families.

In mainstream US culture, where the biomedical explanatory model predominates, child development and behavior are believed to result from a combination of genetic and environmental factors.[22] In the cross-cultural setting, this viewpoint may not be shared by members of an immigrant family, because "patient–provider interactions are complicated by the existence of parallel, usually discrepant, explanatory systems."[23,24] Two tools are useful in exposing differences in explanatory assumptions between cultures: Kleinman's Questions[20] and the LEARN model[25] (**Boxes 2** and **3**). Asking family members what they believe is happening and what causes it is a simple and powerful way to step outside of the ethnocentric assumptions that can create confusion.

Clinical Pearl: Do not assume immigrant families share your explanatory model for a child's development and behavior. Ask them in a nonjudgmental way about their views.

Acculturation gaps between immigrant children and their parents can create a cross-cultural dynamic in the clinical setting that is multidirectional: between provider and parents, provider and patient, and patient and parents. There also can be cultural differences between the nuclear family and extended family members (eg, grandparents), causing disagreement about what is causing a specific problem or even whether it is a problem at all. Asking the family and child about these gaps is critical to understanding how the provider should interact with different family members and how to understand cross-cultural issues in the home. After hearing what a parent thinks about a behavioral or developmental concern, a provider could ask: "Does everyone in the family agree that this is a problem? Does anyone else in the family have other ideas of what might be happening?"

Clinical Pearl: Immigrant families are not homogeneous cultural units; acculturation gaps and generational differences create multidirectional cross-cultural dynamics that should be explored.

Working with Multiple Languages

Language differences make working with interpreters integral to effective communication with immigrant families. Although interpreter use may seem straightforward, it can be complicated in practice, particularly in the pediatric setting. Parents may refuse an interpreter and indicate the child will interpret, or a provider may decide that talking with an adolescent in English is sufficient, especially if a parent speaks or understands a little English. The provider should respectfully explain that children should not be used as interpreters for health care interactions because they lack the vocabulary and developmental capacity needed for health care interpretation. Although adolescents may seem better-equipped to handle this role, only with professionally trained medical interpreters can the provider guarantee that health care language skills and ethical commitment to complete and confidential interpretation will occur.

Box 2
Kleinman's Questions, from the explanatory models approach

What do you call this problem?

What course do you expect it to take? How serious is it?

What do you think this problem does inside your (child's) body?

How does it affect your (child's) body and your (child's) mind?

What do you most fear about this condition?

What do you most fear about the treatment?

What do you believe is the cause of this problem?

Adapted from Kleinman A, Benson P. Anthropology in the clinic: the problem of cultural competency and how to fix it. PLoS Med 2006;3(10):1674; with permission.

Box 3
The LEARN model for cross-cultural communication

L - Listen with sympathy and understanding to the patient's perception of the problem

E - Explain your perception of the problem

A - Acknowledge and discuss the differences and similarities

R - Recommend treatment

N - Negotiate agreement

Adapted from Berlin EA, Fowles WC. A teaching framework for cross-cultural health care: application in family practice. West J Med 1983;139:934.

Discussion of the risks of child interpretation provides an opportunity to review the child's role in the family as language and cultural broker. The role of broker can provide a positive sense of bicultural ability and identity, but also may seem burdensome to a child and may lead to confusing or dangerous situations if the child is required to interpret in high-risk situations (eg, medical, legal).[26,27] Reinforcing the benefits of having children help an immigrant family navigate cross-cultural situations should be balanced with a discussion of the potential risks.

The context of the immigrant family's or child's migration also affects communication. Immigrant families and interpreters may not come from the same country or may come from different classes or castes within a country. Refugees, especially, may come from an ethnic minority that is oppressed in their home country. In such situations, the family and interpreter may use language in different ways and cultural expectations or positions may prevent effective communication. The provider should be alert to signs that there are communication problems, such as long side conversations between the patient and the interpreter, answers that do not make sense, or body language indicating confusion or discomfort. When concerns arise, it is always appropriate to stop and ask for clarification.

Clinical pearl: Begin the visit by asking the interpreter what language he or she is speaking with the family. Ask each family member present (including the child) their preferred language of communication.

Social History Within a Cultural Context

It is helpful to learn a few basic customs related to the culture of the family before beginning the interview. Before entering the room, interpreters can be asked about recommendations on greeting the family, physical interaction and eye contact, and discussion of sensitive topics (eg, trauma, sexual history). World Wide Web–based resources, such as EthnoMed[28] and the Centers for Disease Control and Prevention refugee health profiles,[29] also provide cultural profiles to orient the provider to unfamiliar cultures, including common health beliefs and needs.

A comprehensive social history using the cultural-ecological model of development as a framework can highlight the unique set of factors influencing an immigrant child's development. Such a history should include child characteristics, family context, migration context, settlement context, and ethnic identification (**Box 4**). As for all children, the immigrant child's social history can aid the provider in identifying family strengths, areas of concern, and appropriate referrals. Many immigrant populations are at high risk of developmental delay because of history of trauma, poverty status, and language barriers. Despite this fact, some studies have found an "immigrant advantage" in the areas of social and emotional development, although this depends

---

Box 4
Social history questions from the cultural-ecological perspective

Child Characteristics

Where was the child born?

At what age did the child migrate?

What has the child's school experience been?

Is the child comfortable speaking and reading English?

Is the child comfortable speaking and reading their heritage language?

How does the child feel about being in (host country)?

Family Context

Where were the child's parents born?

Who lives at home? Are there other family members living nearby?

Who in the family has paid work?

What language is spoken at home most of the time?

Are children expected to interpret or translate for their parents? In what situations?

Who in the family speaks or reads English?

Migration Context

How long has the child been in (current city)?

Why did the child/family come to (host country)?

How did the child/family get to (host country)? Did the family all come together?

Are there family members still in (country of origin)?

Settlement Context

Did the family settle in a community of other immigrants?

Do the parents or child feel they are welcomed in their community?

Is the family concerned about Immigrant laws or how the authorities view the family?

Has the child or family experienced discrimination?

Ethnic Identification

What language does the child prefer to speak at home? With friends?

Does the child identify with a race or ethnicity (starting in preadolescence)? If so, which one(s)?

Do parental and child ideas of the child's racial/ethnic identity agree?

---

on many factors (eg, generation of immigrant, parenting practices).[30,31] This has been attributed in part to first-generation children being more likely to live in households where parents are married.[32]

Developmental Surveillance and Screening

The AAP recommends routine developmental screening for all children at the 9-, 18-, and 30-month visits, in addition to developmental surveillance at every visit.[33] Although the recommendation includes children who speak a language other than English, such children are referred for evaluation and intervention at lower rates than their English-speaking counterparts.[34,35] This may be caused in part by the linguistic and cultural challenges of performing developmental screening and surveillance in this group.

There are few translated developmental screens and a wide variation in the evidence for their linguistic and cultural validity.[36] Sensitivity and specificity of validated screening tools vary when used in different cultures than those in which they were originally normed.[37] Even when a translated tool is available, caregivers and patients may have low literacy in their primary language, making completion of a written translated tool impossible. Although it is resource-intensive to have staff read the developmental screener to the family using an interpreter, an advantage to this approach is the ability of the interpreter to ask for further clarification when caregivers have difficulty with the questions. Clinic staff can be alert to the body language and details of answers to assess potential cultural misunderstanding. Further research is needed to determine the most effective way to use screening tools in the multicultural setting. In the meantime, it is important to use existing tools thoughtfully, remembering that they were created from a specific ethnocentric viewpoint and may give discrepant results across cultures. Examples of cultural considerations in developmental screening are presented in **Fig. 5**.

Clinical Pearl: When possible, leave extra time for developmental screening and surveillance with families who do not speak the same language as the provider.

SUPPORTING CHILD DEVELOPMENT IN IMMIGRANT FAMILIES
Bilingualism

In the United States, most children in immigrant families live with a family member who speaks a language other than English at home.[38] Sharing anticipatory guidance, including the benefits of bilingualism, with families of immigrant children provides an opportunity to support and encourage DLLs. Providers should start by acknowledging the strengths conveyed by bilingualism. Bilingual individuals have an advantage on tasks requiring selective attention and cognitive flexibility, with children who receive systematic learning opportunities in their home language during their early years consistently outperforming those who attend English-only classes.[39] Because developing advanced bilingual proficiency requires continued and extensive practice, clinicians should encourage families to share books, sing, and play with their young child frequently in their native language.

Children in immigrant families are much less likely to be growing up in households where there is daily book sharing.[40] Participation in such programs as Reach Out and Read has been shown to improve receptive and expressive language skills and increase the frequency of reading with children.[41,42] Providers should explore cultural beliefs about book sharing and encourage parents to share books daily, regardless of their own literacy level.

When talking to the immigrant child, pointing out that having two languages is a gift, or even a "super power," can help them establish a sense of special ability. Adolescents sometimes are disinterested in maintaining their heritage language. Exploring their resistance should be done with an understanding of how they might be teased, bullied, or otherwise treated badly because of their ethnicity or culture. They may have strong motivation to leave signs of this difference behind as they acculturate into mainstream culture.

Clinical Pearl: Bilingual language development is not a cause for delay of speech acquisition, although there may be qualitative differences in the speech production of bilingual children. Immigrant children with delayed or disordered speech should always be referred.

School/Pre-School/Childcare

Facilities:

✓ Are assessment tools valid for this cultural group?

✓ Are interpreters available?

✓ Do schools have adequate financial resources to address child's needs?

✓ Are teachers/staff able to recognize the signs of developmental delay?

Families/Children:

✓ Do family members recognize signs of developmental delay?

✓ What are their beliefs and attitudes towards developmental delay and screening?

✓ What is the family's background? (SES, education level, urban vs. rural origin, length of residence in the U.S., partnership status, English proficiency, etc.)

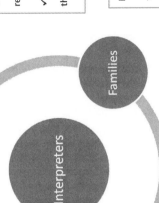

Interpreters:

✓ Is the interpreter knowledgeable about developmental screening?

✓ Is an interpreter available?

✓ What role does the interpreter play? (Social worker, cultural mediator, advocate, etc.)

Pediatricians/Primary Care

Physicians:

✓ Are health care providers trained to conduct developmental screening?

✓ Are screening tools available in target language?

✓ Are the tools culturally appropriate?

✓ Is communication effective among health care provider, interpreter and patient family?

Fig. 5. Cultural considerations in developmental screening. SES, socioeconomic status. (*From* Martin-Herz SP, Kemper T, Brownstein M, et al. Developmental screening with recent immigrant and refugee children: a preliminary report. EthnoMed 2012. Available at: https://ethnomed.org/clinical/pediatrics/developmental-screening-with-recent-immigrant-and-refugee-children. Accessed April 1, 2016; with permission.)

Child Care and School Settings

Although enrollment in high-quality, center-based child care has been shown to improve school readiness in low-income, immigrant children,[43] are enrolled at consistently lower rates than children from nonimmigrant families.[32] Begin to talk with families about benefits of preschool 1 to 2 years before enrollment time, because they may be unfamiliar with the concept of sending young children to school and unaware of enrollment deadlines.

Despite the cognitive and behavioral benefits of bilingualism, there are considerable academic achievement gaps between DLLs (especially Spanish speakers) in the United States and their English-speaking peers.[18] These gaps have spurred innovation in language approaches at schools, with multiple evaluations comparing English-immersion and bilingual methods.[18] Evidence suggests that the latter leads to the best test results, although no consensus has been reached yet about a single best model. Awareness of this debate may help the provider counsel families making decisions about school placement.

Clinical Pearl: Immigrant parents may be unaware of their right to request an evaluation for an individualized family service plan or individualized education program for their child with developmental or learning challenges. Writing down the request in English for them may help bridge any communication gap they may have with school personnel.

Behavioral Disorders/Mental Health

Providers may be asked by parents or teachers to evaluate children from other cultures for developmental or behavioral disorders, such as attention-deficit/hyperactivity disorder or autism. Often parents report school personnel's concerns to providers, although they may not share these concerns. By better understanding the culture of the child's heritage country and the parent's beliefs about child development, the provider is able to more effectively perform these evaluations. For example, in some cultures children are expected to be much more active and tactile with people, and parents may believe behavior defined as hyperactivity and impulsivity in US schools is typical age-appropriate behavior. The provider may help serve as a bridge between school personnel and the family to help both have realistic expectations for integration within the new culture.

Screening for Autism Spectrum Disorder

Autism spectrum disorder (ASD) is characterized by deficits in social and emotional communication and behavior.[44] The core components of ASD require interpretation within a cultural context, so challenges in appropriate diagnosis and treatment are inevitable. In February 2016, the US Preventive Services Task Force concluded that current evidence is insufficient to assess the balance of benefits and harms of screening for ASD in young children for whom no concerns of ASD have been raised by their parents or a clinician.[45] The AAP issued an immediate response standing behind their recommendation to screen all children at 18 and 24 months.[46] Given the challenges of developmental surveillance in children from immigrant families, including linguistic/cultural differences and parent expectations for typical behavior, we recommend universal screening for immigrant children in addition to routine surveillance.

Research on how culture and language relate to autism has increased dramatically in the last decade with the increase in prevalence of ASD. Prevalence has been found to vary by race and ethnicity, with lower rates but more severe symptoms in Latino and African American children.[47] Autism prevalence in the Somali population in Minneapolis was recently found to be 1 in 32 in 7- to 9-year old children.[48] This was similar to the prevalence in white children, but higher than non-Somali black children or Latino children. Somali children had more severe intellectual disability at the time of diagnosis.

Maternal nativity and ethnicity were recently found to be a risk factor for ASD in US populations.[47] Compared with children of US-born white mothers, those whose mothers were foreign-born black, Central/South American, Filipino, and Vietnamese, or US-born African American and Latino mothers, had a higher risk of severe autism phenotypes. The role of genetics in autism is only beginning to be understood, and the intersection of genetics, ethnicity, and culture is an area ripe with research opportunities.

Clinical Pearl: Be vigilant about the possibility of ASD in children in immigrant families with language delay. Bilingualism (or monolingualism in the heritage language) and cultural beliefs make detection of ASD difficult in the context of a primary care visit. When in doubt, refer to appropriate birth to age 3 screening services, available in every state.

Trauma

Migration context, including history of trauma, is an important consideration for mental health referrals. The process of migration involves varying levels of trauma. A child with highly educated parents who speak English migrating for well-paid work may experience the trauma of leaving family and friends. This child's migration experience is different from that of a former child soldier who witnessed and committed violence and migrated as a refugee. No matter the migration and settlement contexts, a trauma-informed approach to clinical care is essential during initial evaluation and on-going care.

According to the Substance Abuse and Mental Health Administration, "a program, organization, or system that is trauma-informed: 1. Realizes the widespread impact of trauma and understands potential paths for recovery; 2. Recognizes the signs and symptoms of trauma in clients, families, staff, and others involved with the system; 3. Responds by fully integrating knowledge about trauma into policies, procedures, and practices; and 4. Seeks to actively resist re-traumatization."[49] The AAP Trauma Toolbox, developed for pediatricians in the primary care setting, offers specific guidelines on caring for children and families who have experienced trauma.[50]

Refugee children have a heightened risk for severe trauma, which can have profound effects on their emotional, mental, and physical health.[51] When working with refugee children, in addition to seeking specialist support, providers can find guidance in the Refugee Services Toolkit from the National Child Traumatic Stress Network, created to help service system providers understand the experience of refugee children and families, identify the needs associated with their mental health, and ensure they are connected with the most appropriate available interventions.[52]

Poverty

Screening and appropriate referrals for families living in poverty is an important way to support children living in immigrant families, who are more likely to live in low-income households with parents without a high school degree.[39] Keep a list of culturally sensitive resource providers for immigrant families and discuss with clinic-based social workers their approach to immigrant families from frequently encountered cultures.

Legal Issues

Legal issues are a significant stressor for children in immigrant families and a frequent question at primary care provider visits. Separation from one or both parents and other family members because of partial family immigration or deportation has become a common experience for immigrant children, described as one of the most difficult aspects of immigrating.[53] In addition to evaluating the effect family separations or reunifications might have on the immigrant child, the provider may be asked to provide information to the family for immigration proceedings. Guidance on ways to respond are found in the AAP Immigrant Health Toolkit.[4] The US federal government also provides a list of free immigration legal services by state on the Department of Justice Web site,[54] with information on immigration scams and disciplined immigration attorneys on the US Citizenship and Immigration Services Web site.[55]

For refugee children, the Office of Refugee Resettlement provides time-limited cash and medical assistance to new arrivals to help them attain self-sufficiency. The first 8 months after a refugee arrives in this country, they are covered by Refugee Medicaid, so this is a critical time for identifying health problems, including issues that may affect development, such as vitamin deficiencies, elevated lead levels, poor vision or hearing, parasitic infections, and so forth. The Office of Refugee Resettlement also offers a policy guide to aid providers in the care of unaccompanied immigrant children.[56]

SUMMARY

As the United States moves toward a majority-minority future, where a third of children will have at least one foreign-born parent, the engagement of child health researchers and clinicians in the affairs of immigrant families will be critical to providing the highest quality care to a population at heightened risk of being misunderstood and misdiagnosed. Although there are numerous developmental models and tools available to the practicing provider, many of them have yet to be fully adapted for use with children of immigrant families. As research continues to fill gaps in knowledge and practice, awareness of the known developmental benefits and risks related to immigration can help the pediatrician develop a clinical approach that is appropriate for each child. No matter the pediatrician's level of experience with immigrant families, most essential to success in the cross-cultural setting is a stance of cultural humility, from which the provider can overcome obstacles to excellent communication, care, and outcomes.

REFERENCES

1. Federal interagency forum on child and family statistics. America's children: key national indicators of well-being, 2015. "Children of at least one foreign born parent." Available at: http://www.childstats.gov/americaschildren/family4.asp. Accessed March 25, 2016.
2. Passel JS. Demography of immigrant youth: past, present, and future. Future Child 2011;21(1):19–41.
3. Office of Refugee Resettlement. Refugee arrival data FY2104. Available at: http://www.acf.hhs.gov/programs/orr/resource/refugee-arrival-data. Accessed March 30, 2016.
4. American Academy of Pediatrics. Immigrant child health toolkit. Available at: https://www.aap.org/en-us/about-the-aap/Committees-Councils-Sections/Council-on-Community-Pediatrics/Pages/Immigrant-Child-Health-Toolkit.aspx. Accessed March 30, 2016.
5. Linton JM, Choi R, Mendoza F. Caring for children in immigrant families: vulnerabilities, resilience, and opportunities. Pediatr Clin North Am 2016;63(1):115–30.
6. Bronfenbrenner U. The ecology of human development: experiments by nature and design. Cambridge (MA): Harvard University Press; 1979.

7. Perreira KM, Smith L. A cultural-ecological model of migration and development: focusing on Latino immigrant youth. Prev Res 2007;14(4):6–9.
8. Suárez-Orozco C, Abo-Zena MM, Marks AK. Transitions: the development of the children of immigrants. New York: New York University Press; 2015.
9. Berry JW. Immigration, acculturation, and adaptation. Appl Psychol 1997;46(1):5–34.
10. Bourhis RY, Moise LC, Perreault S, et al. Towards an interactive acculturation model: a social psychological approach. Int J Psychol 1997;32(6):369–86.
11. Birman D, Addae D. Acculturation. In: Suárez-Orozco C, Abo-Zena MM, Marks AK, editors. Transitions: the development of the children of immigrants. New York: NYU Press; 2015. p. 122–41.
12. Schwartz SJ, Cano MA, Zamboanga BL. Identity development. In: Suárez-Orozco C, Abo-Zena MM, Marks AK, editors. Transitions: the development of the children of immigrants. New York: NYU Press; 2015. p. 142–64.
13. Huynh QL, Devos T, Smalarz L. Perpetual foreigner in one's own land: potential implications for identity and psychological adjustment. J Soc Clin Psychol 2011;30(2):133–62.
14. Kovács ÁM. Cognitive adaptations induced by a multi-language input in early development. Curr Opin Neurobiol 2015;35:80–6.
15. Wong B, Yin B, O'Brien B. Neurolinguistics: structure, function, and connectivity in the bilingual brain. Biomed Res Int 2016;2016:1–22.
16. Barac R, Bialystok E, Castro DC, et al. The cognitive development of young dual language learners: a critical review. Early Child Res Q 2014;29(4):699–714.
17. Halle TG, Whittaker JV, Zepeda M, et al. The social-emotional development of dual language learners: looking back at existing research and moving forward with purpose. Early Child Res Q 2014;29(4):734–49.
18. Páez MM, Hunter CJ. Bilingualism and language learning. In: Suárez-Orozco C, Abo-Zena MM, Marks AK, editors. Transitions: the development of the children of immigrants. New York: NYU Press; 2015. p. 165–83.
19. Onchwari G, Onchwari JA, Keengwe J. Teaching the immigrant child: application of child development theories. Early Child Educ J 2008;36:267–73.
20. Kleinman A, Benson P. Anthropology in the clinic: the problem of cultural competency and how to fix it. PLoS Med 2006;3(10):1673–6.
21. US Department of Health and Human Services, Office of Minority Health. National Standards for Culturally and Linguistically Appropriate Services (CLAS) in Health and Health Care. Available at: https://www.thinkculturalhealth.hhs.gov/content/clas.asp. Accessed March 25, 2016.
22. National Research Council (US), Institute of Medicine (US). Children's health, the nation's wealth: assessing and improving child health. Washington, DC: National Academies Press; 2004. p. 3. Influences on Children's Health. Available at: http://www.ncbi.nlm.nih.gov/books/NBK92200/. Accessed April 2, 2016.
23. Melendez L. Parental beliefs and practices around early self-regulation: the impact of culture and immigration. Infants Young Child 2005;18(2):136–46.
24. Putsch RW, Joyce M. Dealing with patients from other cultures. In: Walker HK, Hall WD, Hurst JW, editors. Clinical methods: the history, physical, and laboratory examinations. 3rd edition. Boston: Butterworths; 1990. p. 1050–9.
25. Berlin EA, Fowles WC. A teaching framework for cross-cultural health care: application in family practice. West J Med 1983;139:934–8.
26. Flores G, Abreu M, Barone CP, et al. Errors of medical interpretation and their potential clinical consequences: a comparison of professional versus ad hoc versus no interpreters. Ann Emerg Med 2012;60(5):545–53.

27. Juckett G, Unger K. Appropriate use of medical interpreters. Am Fam Physician 2014;90(7):476–80.

28. EthnoMed. Available at: https://ehtnomed.org. Accessed March 30, 2016.

29. Centers for Disease Control and Prevention (CDC). Refugees Health Profiles. Available at: http://www.cdc.gov/immigrantrefugeehealth/profiles. Accessed March 30, 2016.

30. De Feyter JJ, Winsler A. The early developmental competencies and school readiness of low-income, immigrant children: influences of generation, race/ethnicity, and national origins. Early Child Res Q 2009;24:411–31.

31. Chun H, Mobley M. The "immigrant paradox" phenomenon: assessing problem behaviors and risk factors among immigrant and native adolescents. J Prim Prev 2014;35(5):339–56.

32. Child Trends. Data Bank. Immigrant children: indicators on children and youth. 2014. Available at: http://www.childtrends.org/?indicators=immigrant-children. Accessed April 1, 2016.

33. American Academy of Pediatrics. Policy statement: identifying infants and young children with developmental disorders in the medical home: an algorithm for developmental surveillance and screening. Pediatrics 2006;118(1): 405–20.

34. Mandell DS, Listerud J, Levy SE, et al. Race differences in the age at diagnosis among Medicaid-eligible children with autism. J Am Acad Child Adolesc Psychiatry 2002;41:1447–53.

35. Beeger S, El Bouk S, Boussaid W, et al. Underdiagnosis and referral bias of autism in ethnic minorities. J Autism Dev Disord 2009;39:142–8.

36. El-Behadli AF, Neger EN, Perrin EC, et al. Translations of developmental screening instruments: an evidence map of available research. J Dev Behav Pediatr 2015;36(6):471–83.

37. Geddes JS. Measuring early childhood development in refugee children [master's thesis]. Perth (Australia): University of Western Australia; 2012.

38. Capps R, Fix M, Ost J, et al. The health and well-being of young children of immigrants. Washington, DC: The Urban Institute; 2004.

39. Espinosa LM. Challenging common myths about dual language learners, an update to the seminal 2008 report. PreK-3rd Policy Action Brief. New York: Foundation for Child Development; 2013.

40. Festa N, Loftus PD, Cullen MR, et al. Disparities in early exposure to book sharing within immigrant families. Pediatrics 2014;134:e162–168.

41. Mendelsohn AL, Mogilner LN, Dreyer BP, et al. The impact of a clinic-based literacy intervention on language development in inner-city preschool children. Pediatrics 2001;107:130–4.

42. Needlman R, Toker KH, Dreyer BP, et al. Effectiveness of a primary care intervention to support reading aloud: a multicenter evaluation. Ambul Pediatr 2005;5(4): 209–15.

43. Burchinal M, Vandergrift N, Pianta R, et al. Threshold analysis of association between child care quality and child outcomes for low-income children in prekindergarten programs. Early Child Res Q 2009;25:166–76.

44. American Psychiatric Association. Diagnostic and statistical manual of mental disorders. 5th edition. Arlington (VA): American Psychiatric Publishing; 2013.

45. Siu AL, US Preventive Services Task Force (USPSTF). Screening for autism spectrum disorder in young children: US Preventive Services Task Force statement. JAMA 2016;315(7):691–6.

46. Dreyer BP. AAP statement on U.S. preventive services task force final recommendation statement on autism screening. 2016. Available at: https://www.aap.org/en-us/about-the-aap/aap-press-room/Pages/AAP-Statement-on-US-Preventive-Services-Task-Force-Final-Recommendation-Statement-on-Autism-Screening.aspx. Accessed March 15, 2016.

47. Becerra TA, von Ehrenstein OS, Heck JE, et al. Autism spectrum disorders and race, ethnicity, and nativity: a population-based study. Pediatrics 2014;134(1): e63–71.

48. Hewitt A, Gulaid A, Hamre K, et al. Minneapolis Somali autism spectrum disorder prevalence project: community report 2013. Minneapolis (MN): University of Minnesota, Institute on Community Integration, Research and Training Center on Community Living; 2013.

49. Substance Abuse and Mental Health Administration (SAMHSA). Trauma-informed approach and trauma-specific interventions. Available at: http://www.samhsa.gov/nctic/trauma-interventions. Accessed March 9, 2016.

50. American Academy of Pediatrics. Trauma guide. Available at: https://www.aap.org/en- us/advocacy-and-policy/aap-health-initiatives/healthy-foster-care- america/Pages/Trauma-Guide.aspx#trauma. Accessed March 15, 2016.

51. Tam SY, Houlihan S, Melendez-Torres GJ. A systematic review of longitudinal risk and protective factors and correlates for posttraumatic stress and its natural history in forcibly displaced children. Trauma Violence Abuse 2015. [Epub ahead of print].

52. National Child Traumatic Stress Network (NCTSN). Refugee services toolkit. Available at: http://learn.nctsn.org/course/view.php?id=62. Accessed April 1, 2016.

53. Suárez-Orozco C. Family separations and reunifications. In: Suárez-Orozco C, Abo-Zena MM, Marks AK, editors. Transitions: the development of the children of immigrants. New York: NYU Press; 2015. p. 32–46.

54. US Department of Justice. Executive office for immigration review. List of pro bono legal service advisors. Available at: https://www.justice.gov/eoir/list-pro-bono-legal-service-providers. Accessed March 31, 2016.

55. US Citizenship and Immigration Services. Immigration and Nationality Act Web site. Available at: https://www.uscis.gov/laws/immigration-and-nationality-act. Accessed March 31, 2016.

56. US Office of Refugee Resettlement. Unaccompanied Children's Services. Available at: http://www.acf.hhs.gov/programs/orr/programs/ucs. Accessed March 31, 2016.

Impact of Military Deployment on the Development and Behavior of Children

Suzie C. Nelson, MD*, Matthew J. Baker, DO,
Christina G. Weston, MD

KEYWORDS

- Military children • Deployment • Child development • Child behavior • Family risk

KEY POINTS

- Military culture has changed in recent years, increasing the likelihood that military-connected children will be affected by stresses unique to military life.
- Military deployment, resulting in separation of parents from their families for long periods of time, has repercussions on child development and behavior.
- Interventions to strengthen family resilience and parenting skills/coping have shown promise in mitigating potentially negative outcomes following deployment.
- More research, including longitudinal studies of military families, is needed to design further interventions and to bolster policies that support military families.

INTRODUCTION

In 1973, the US military initiated a significant shift within its own culture, transitioning from a draft force to an all-volunteer force (AVF), and consequently the lives of military families has gained increasing importance in military policy. Before this time, most who embraced the military as a lifelong career tended to be senior military service members, with most of the force consisting of young, unmarried men who served a tour and transitioned to civilian life before beginning a family. With the introduction of the AVF, larger groups of younger service members joined and remained in the military, and the growing population of junior military service members began families and

Disclosures: The authors have no conflict of interest. The views expressed in this article are those of the authors and do not reflect the official policy or position of the Department of the Army, Navy, Air Force, Defense, or the US Government.
Department of Psychiatry, Wright State University Boonshoft School of Medicine, 627 South Edwin C. Moses Boulevard, Dayton, OH 45417-1461, USA
* Corresponding author.
E-mail address: suzie.nelson@wright.edu

Pediatr Clin N Am 63 (2016) 795–811
http://dx.doi.org/10.1016/j.pcl.2016.06.003
0031-3955/16/$ – see front matter Published by Elsevier Inc.

pediatric.theclinics.com

chose the military as a career.[1] The AVF military has seen the longest sustained deployment of service members to Afghanistan and Iraq[2]; consequently, deployment has become a way of life for military families, with stateside family members serving the military in their own unique ways. The welfare of military families has gained attention at the nation's highest levels with President Obama declaring "the care and support of military families a top national security policy priority."[3]

Provision of this care occurs in medical and mental health practices across the country. The scope of clinical practice involving military-connected children is broad, because of the widespread presence of military families in communities across the United States, many of which do not surround military installations. For the purposes of this article, the military family is defined as the spouses and dependent children of active duty (AD), National Guard, and Reserve military service members; many of the available studies involve current military-connected children, although the authors recognize that there are many other affected families of military veterans.

MILITARY CULTURE
Demographics

With the growing number of military service members remaining on AD while they begin families, military family members outnumber military personnel by 1.36 to 1, and there is a growing diversity of family forms. In 2014, 665,619 spouses and more than 1.12 million dependent children lived in AD families, and 381,773 spouses and 699,835 dependent children lived in Guard and Reserve families. Another 2 million children are dependents of veterans, bringing the total number of military-connected children to 4 million.[4]

Some specific financial and social circumstances create an environment in which military members are more likely to be married and to have children at younger ages compared with civilian counterparts. Almost all military service members have high job security for a contracted service commitment typically lasting a few years, and active military members have higher income levels than civilian counterparts in many career fields.[5] Increased housing allowance following marriage, the presence of stable health care for the entire family, and the provision of quality day care and other family support services all remove some of the potential financial barriers to beginning a family at younger ages.[6] The military tends to draw people with conservative family values, thus increasing the likelihood that those involved in the military will marry and begin families at younger ages, as well.[7] For those services in which most of the force is young, such as the Marine Corps, service members marry at younger ages and have children of younger ages. In contrast, in the Air Force and Navy the organizational culture tends to value retention of experience and more advanced technological training; thus, a greater proportion of these service members tends to be older and have older children. Overall, military-connected children are younger, with the largest group between birth and 5 years of age (**Fig. 1**).[4]

School and Family Life

About 13% of children of AD parents attend Department of Defense Education Activity schools, in the United States and overseas. The remainder attend civilian schools in communities surrounding military bases.[8] Many children of AD parents are concentrated near enough to a large military base to attend schools with staff who are familiar with military culture and have an awareness of their unique needs. However, those located far away from military bases typically attend schools and live in communities

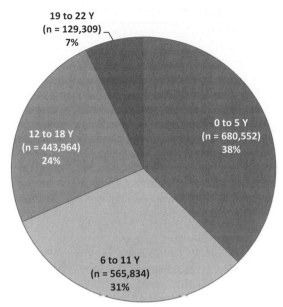

19 to 22 Y
(n = 129,309)
7%

0 to 5 Y
(n = 680,552)
38%

12 to 18 Y
(n = 443,964)
24%

6 to 11 Y
(n = 565,834)
31%

Fig. 1. Age of military children (N = 1,819,659). Children aged 21 to 22 years must be enrolled as full-time students in order to qualify as dependents. Percentages may not total 100 because of rounding. (*From* Passel JS. Demography of immigrant youth: past, present, and future. Future Child 2011;21(1):19–41, with permission.)

that have less experience working with military families; these families face the dual challenges of decreased awareness of military cultural factors in their own communities and also of being separated from the resources near military bases. According to the Citizen Soldier Support Program, all but 12 counties in the United States were home to at least 1 of the 1.3 million Reserve members serving in 2012.[9] Thus, a large number of military-connected children may be struggling with deployment-related family adjustments and also lacking access to base resources and military community connections.

For AD families, there are dual-service challenges for those led by 2 active-duty parents: even though there may be efforts to keep these families together, staffing needs may require them to live in different areas of the United States or even endure an overseas separation. In these cases, a difficult decision about where the children will live must be made. Single parents who are on AD face challenges inherent to single parenthood in any community, but many single civilian parents live near extended family networks, a choice not always available at the military base at which the service member is stationed. Single parents and dual-military parent families must also have a care plan in place should the need for training or deployment require parents to be away from their children for extended periods of time.[10] Still other families, in which there is 1 AD parent and 1 civilian parent, must endure separations because of the difficult choice between allowing a child to have academic and social stability, or, because of financial constraints, preventing the family from moving with the AD member. These circumstances increase the likelihood that military families will face separations of parents from children, not only during a deployment but also at other times and for long durations.

Relocation

Over the course of a family's time associated with the military, it is likely they will face at least 1 move outside the continental United States and the deployment of a parent. Compared with civilian families, AD military families move 2.4 times as often, with relocation occurring every 2 to 3 years, and over long distances, across state lines, or to foreign countries.[11] By contrast, Guard and Reserve families have relocation patterns comparable with those of civilian families.

Identity and Resilience

Military families face many adversities caused by the requirements of military life, including multiple moves, changing schools and social networks, parental deployments, reintegration, and the potential dangers for injury or even death of the service member. However, these families also share a common identity of strength and sacrifice, and the special meaning of service to country is a significant resilience factor that is not only immediately protective but also probably contributes to the increased likelihood that children of service members will go on to choose a career in the military themselves.[12] Characteristics unique to military life create both opportunities to promote resilience in children and potential challenges to healthy childhood development and behavior.

DEVELOPMENTAL REVIEW

To better understand the impact of a significant family event, such as the deployment of a military parent, on child development, an overview of some basic concepts from both childhood and family psychological development is important.

Attachment

The work of Margaret Mahler and Mary Ainsworth emphasizes the importance of what is classically described as the mother-infant dyad, although the authors recognize that the mother can also be another caregiver who is the primary attachment figure for the child. Insecure attachment styles predict greater difficulty with peer relationships, emotional self-regulation, and school adjustment and functioning. By contrast, secure attachments arise out of the parent's ability to discern, accept, and interpret the infant's emotional needs. In this sense, secure attachments are born of the parent's ability to be an external source of emotional regulation for the child. Secure attachments are protective for the child emotionally, cognitively, socially, and physically.[13] With the potential for impact from the physical absence of a parent during later stages of infancy, and with the potential distress on the caregiving parent left at home, management of stress for the caregiving parent during the other parent's extended absence can be an important factor in fostering secure attachments in this population. This factor prepares for greater resilience for these children as their families navigate military life. Because critical periods of development throughout childhood and adolescence arguably manifest out of the responsiveness of a parent to a child's emotional needs, the ability of a caregiving parent to be present for the child is of considerable importance. This ability is especially important during stressful family events such as the other parent's deployment; if there are more routine family changes, such as moving across the country; and in the event of extraordinary circumstances such as the death or significant injury of a parent during combat.

Family Functioning and Systems Theory

Functional families are characterized by parents who give children the emotional room to learn, interact with peer groups, form an identity, and acquire responsibility and maturity themselves. Military families do not differ in needing these characteristics to function well, but certain ones are of special consideration because of differences in military culture. Adaptability to external demands is essential, potentially on a repeated basis, because the military regularly requires much flexibility from its families in the form of multiple moves and multiple family member separations. Likewise, having adequate resources in the form of community and social networks, which for a military family continually change with each relocation, is vital to allow family members to thrive. Family systems theory teaches that each member of a family interacts with the other family members in ways that influence all of the relationships; likewise, military families also operate within the military as a system. Changes within individual family members (internal) and changes caused by the requirements of the military (external) all have ripple effects within the family.[14]

THE DEPLOYMENT CYCLE

Of significance to military families is the event of the service member's deployment, requiring absence from the family for an extended period of time. Five distinct stages of deployment have been described (**Fig. 2, Table 1**).[15] Each comprises a specific time frame and particular emotional challenges that the military family must successfully navigate to avoid undesirable consequences.

Predeployment begins when the service member and family learn of the impending deployment, and it is characterized by anticipation of separation. The second stage, deployment, proceeds from departure through the first month away and involves an initial adjustment reaction. Sustainment, the third stage, is endured from the first month through the next to the last month of deployment. It is a critical time for the family to create new routines and find new sources of emotional and social support from other family, friends, religious groups, or community groups. Successful navigation of this stage can help the at-home spouse build confidence and a sense of control. Children may take on new responsibilities and independence. Stage 4, redeployment,

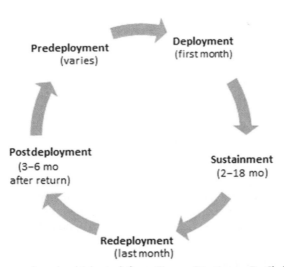

Fig. 2. The deployment cycle. (*Adapted from* Pincus SH, House R, Christenson J, et al. The emotional cycle of deployment: a military family perspective. Available at: http://www.mwrgl.com/child_youth/slo/slo_linkedfiles/EmotionalCycleofDeployment.pdf.)

Table 1
Emotional characteristics by stage of deployment

Predeployment	Deployment	Sustainment	Redeployment	Postdeployment
Denial vs anticipation of loss	Loneliness, sadness	Establishing new supports	Excitement, increased energy	Joy and relief
Fears and worries	Abandonment	New responsibilities	Anticipation of return/reunion	Frustration and tension
Arguments	Disorganization, disorientation	Independence	Ambivalence	Changed responsibilities
Regressive behaviors in children	Disorientation, overwhelmed	Increased or decreased confidence	Apprehension, difficulty making decisions	Altered communication, relationships

Data from Pincus SH, House R, Christenson J, et al. The emotional cycle of deployment: a military family perspective. Available at: http://www.mwrgl.com/child_youth/slo/slo_linkedfiles/Emotional CycleofDeployment.pdf.

pertains to the month before a service member's return home and typically involves feelings of excitement, but it may also be characterized by some ambivalence caused by potential loss of newfound independence and role changes. The final stage, post-deployment, begins with the homecoming of the service member and spans the subsequent 3 to 6 months. Reintegration of the service member into the family can lead to tension as responsibilities are reallocated and reunions are complicated by the possibility that family members, rules, and norms in the home have changed. This final, most critical phase also presents the opportunity for improvements in communication, relationships, and future goals that can build strength and resilience to confront future challenges.[15]

EFFECTS OF DEPLOYMENT ON CHILDREN

Some deployment effects are generalizable to all children, whereas others are specific depending on the child's age. Several excellent reviews have compiled the evidence in recent years.[16–20] Differences that depend on each service (eg, Army, Navy, Air Force, National Guard) are more difficult to determine because of the lack of comparison studies. Although most children seem to function well during the deployment cycle, some experience negative effects that commonly occur during and/or after the deployment.

GENERAL FINDINGS ACROSS CHILDHOOD
Increased Emotional and Behavioral Problems

Parental deployment seems to be associated with increased emotional and behavioral problems among military children, aged 3 to 17 years, compared with community norms, and seems to be most pronounced in older children both during and after deployment.[21,22] Parenting stress and mental health status of the home caregiver seem to be associated with increases in internalizing and externalizing symptoms in their children.[23]

Changes in Health Care Use

Retrospective studies of medical records showed deployment-related changes in health care use. For children aged 3 to 17 years, a direct correlation was found between length of deployment and increasing risk for mental health visits for acute stress reaction, adjustment disorder, depressive disorders, and behavioral disorders.[24] In other studies examining a less broad age range, general findings included an increased rate of specialty care visits, especially those that were mental health related,[25,26] but a decrease in overall health care visits. Reasons for increasing visits tended to include general mental health complaints, injuries, child maltreatment,[27] and increased visits for preexisting mental health conditions, such as attention-deficit/hyperactivity disorder.[28] In addition, there were increased rates of antidepressant (17.2%) and antianxiety (10%) prescriptions.[26]

Increased Child Maltreatment

AD Army families experienced a 42% increase in the rate of child maltreatment during parental deployment, particularly rates of moderate to severe maltreatment. The level of neglect nearly doubled, whereas emotional and physical abuse seemed to decrease during deployment.[29] Rates of severe maltreatment may be higher following a combat deployment, especially when involving alcohol use.[30] Another study similarly found that rates of child maltreatment doubled during deployment, with increases around the times of service member departure and return; the rates were highest in children less than 4 years of age. Military families seemed to have less overall maltreatment than nonmilitary families,[31] implying that there are certain stabilizing factors in military families at baseline that are overcome during deployment.

Decline in School Performance

The effect of deployment on school performance seems to be modest but significant. Findings for grades 3 to 11 in Department of Defense schools showed modest adverse effects in multiple academic subjects if a parent was deployed at some point during the school year, with longer deployments yielding greater effects.[32] Another study found that elementary and middle school students had a modest but significant reduction in achievement scores when a parent had deployed for 19 months or more compared with children with less or no parental deployment.[33]

INFANTS AND TODDLERS
Increased Risk of Preterm Birth and Postpartum Depression

Spousal deployment may be associated with a higher risk of preterm birth,[34] as well as increased risk of postpartum depression,[34,35] although group prenatal care may mitigate this effect.[34]

Disturbances of Attachment and Development

Children whose parents deployed failed measures of social-emotional functioning at twice the rate of children whose parents did not deploy.[36] Children 0 to 47 months old showed signs of attachment strain during a parental deployment: trouble sleeping alone, not seeking comfort from the returned parent, not wanting the returned parent to leave the home, and preferring the nondeployed spouse or caregiver to the returned parent.[37]

Increased Emotional and Behavioral Problems

Measures of internalizing behaviors,[38] rates of sadness among children aged 3 to 5 years,[39] and an 18% increase in stress disorder diagnosis among children aged 3 to 8 years are among the indications of problems with internalizing behaviors within this age group.[25] Alongside these findings, externalizing behaviors were also shown by increased externalizing measures,[38] rates of aggressive behaviors among children aged 3 to 5 years,[39] and a 19% increase in behavior disorder diagnoses among children aged 3 to 8 years.[25]

SCHOOL-AGED CHILDREN
Increased Emotional and Behavioral Problems

Children aged 6 to 12 years had symptoms of anxiety, worry, and sadness that exceeded community norms.[39–41] Both internalizing symptoms, such as depression, and externalizing symptoms were associated with cumulative length of parent combat-related deployment during the child's lifetime, parental distress in both the at-home and AD parents, and symptoms of anxiety and depression in home caregivers. Girls had higher externalizing scores during the deployment, whereas boys showed symptom increases when the parent returned.[41] Parenting stress in AD families was associated with reports of increased child behavior problems on the Pediatric Symptom Checklist, with scores 2.5 times national norms[42]; risks were particularly increased for psychosocial problems, internalizing, externalizing, and inattention symptoms. Perceived support from family, church, nonmilitary organizations, and military organizations helped mitigate family stress. Increased somatic symptoms among school-aged children, which may be linked to anxiety or internalizing symptoms, has also been noted in children during parental deployment.[41,43]

ADOLESCENTS
Increased Emotional and Behavioral Problems

Home caregivers indicated that their adolescent children, aged 11 to 17 years, with a deployed parent had greater emotional difficulties compared with national means; older age of the child, increased length of parental deployment, and poorer mental health of the home caregiver were associated with increased reports of school, family, and peer difficulties during deployment.[44] Adolescents reported increased psychosocial symptoms,[45] as well as difficulty controlling anger.[46] Increased posttraumatic stress disorder symptoms, stress scores, increased heart rates, and higher systolic blood pressures were found in a small sample of adolescents with a deployed parent.[47] Teenagers admit difficulties with emotional stress, worries about the deployed parent, and concerns about caregiver stress when a parent is deployed.[48]

Suicidality

An adolescent youth survey revealed that having a deployed parent increased the risk of suicidal ideation. This finding was accompanied by reports of lower quality of life during the parental deployment and depressed mood. These reports were significantly more common than those by adolescents in civilian or nondeployed military families.[49]

Increased Conduct Problems and Substance Use

A statewide youth survey found that parental deployment was associated with increased reports of gang membership and physical fighting among older adolescents.[49] Increased weapon carrying and victimization by peers were found in adolescents of deployed parents, as well as an association between parental deployment and lifetime use of tobacco or other drugs.[50] Adolescents with a deployed parent were significantly more likely to report binge drinking in the previous 2 weeks compared with civilian adolescents.[51] Similarly, a survey of sixth, eighth, and eleventh graders in Iowa found that children of currently or recently deployed service members had higher reports of drinking alcohol, binge drinking, prescription drug abuse, marijuana use, and other substance use than adolescents from nonmilitary families, with some risks higher if living with someone who was a nonparent.[52]

Decline in School Performance

Adolescents with a deployed parent were concerned about changes in family routines, increased responsibilities, and decreased academic performance.[53] Adolescents 13 to 18 years old seem to have the largest decreases in academic performance during periods of parental deployment.[39] Older teens reported more school and peer problems than younger teens.[54,55] Children 11 to 16 years old with a deployed parent reported more school difficulties than other children.[45]

INTERVENTIONS FOR FAMILIES

Addressing the challenges that military families face when coping with deployment is complex because of the difficulty in providing interventions across a wide geographic area, among different service branches, and with families who may be facing multiple simultaneous stressors at once, such as a returning parent combined with a military move. Studies are often limited to distinct military bases or areas and most do not address needs of Guard and Reserve families. With those limitations noted, a variety of interventions for military families have been proposed, and the small but growing evidence base provides promising results that may be widely applicable in the future. Interventions range from education about the deployment process, to prevention in at-risk populations, to treatment of those with significant mental health problems. The Institute of Medicine has recommended that at-risk and distressed populations be targeted for prevention efforts.[56]

Families Overcoming Under Stress

Families Overcoming Under Stress (FOCUS) was designed as a family-centered program for military families with numerous deployments to enhance resilience and reduce psychological health risk.[57] It combines features from 2 evidence-based family-centered preventive interventions that improve family and child adjustment in the context of parental medical or mental health difficulties,[58,59] along with another intervention for children and parents affected by wartime deployments.[60] This improvement is accomplished through promotion of family functioning via improved parent-parent relationships and parent-child relationships, in addition to provision of individual help when needed for children and/or parents. The success of FOCUS shows that improving family functioning improves individual well-being and vice versa.

Table 2 provides an overview of the core elements of FOCUS.[57] The intervention is delivered via in-person, provider-led sessions for individual families over 8 sessions with a combination of parent-only, child-only, and family sessions. To date, FOCUS has enrolled 2615 families at 15 military installations in the United States and Japan. The families had an average of 4.53 total deployments before enrollment. At completion of the program and 6-month follow-up, parental anxiety and depression were significantly reduced. Both boys and girls showed improvements in emotional and behavioral symptoms and in prosocial behaviors. The investigators also noted improvements in parental anxiety, depression, and posttraumatic stress symptoms.[57] Most participants are enrolled because of proximity to a military base at which FOCUS is offered. In recognition of this limitation, FOCUS developers have created Web-based access to educational materials as well as the interactive family resiliency training for those families not colocated with the available program. Table 3 provides

Table 2
Comparison of FOCUS and ADAPT interventions

	FOCUS	ADAPT
Interventions Provided	Evaluation of family health Provide developmental guidance Parenting psychoeducation Create shared family narrative Teach resilience skills • Goal setting • Problem solving • Communication • Emotional regulation • Management of reminders	Skill encouragement Positive involvement Family problem solving Monitoring Effective discipline Psychoeducation on combat stress
Population	AD military	Guard/Reserve parents
Format	Individual: parent, child and family sessions	Group: parent only
Length	8 sessions	14 sessions

Data from Beardslee W, Lester P, Klosinski L, et al. Family-centered preventive intervention for military families: implications for implementation science. Prev Sci 2011;12(4):339–48; and Gewirtz AH, Pinna KL, Hanson SK, et al. Promoting parenting to support reintegrating military families: after deployment, adaptive parenting tools. Psychol Serv 2014;11(1):31.

a list of Internet resources. The Web site also allows booster training for families who have completed FOCUS.[61]

After Deployment, Adaptive Parenting Tools

Recognition that National Guard and Reserve soldiers have deployed but have limited access to military base services has led to the development of a parenting support

Table 3
Internet resources

Military One Source: online and phone resources for all AD Services, Reserves, and National Guard	www.militaryonesource.com
Tragedy Assistance Program for Survivors: offers assistance for those who have lost a service member	www.tabs.org
American Academy of Pediatrics: resources for pediatricians	https://www.aap.org/en-us/advocacy-and-policy/aap-health-initiatives/Pages/Deployment-and-Military.aspx
VA resources for providers	www.mentalhealth.va.gov/communityproviders/index.asp
Center for Deployment Psychology: online training	http://deploymentpsych.org/
AACAP resources	http://www.aacap.org/AACAP/Families_and_Youth/Resource_Centers/Military_Families_Resource_Center/Home.aspx
Sesame Workshop: military initiatives guide for families with young children	http://www.sesameworkshop.org/what-we-do/our-initiatives/military-families
FOCUS Web site and access to online training modules	http://www.focusproject.org/home

Abbreviation: AACAP, American Academy of Child and Adolescent Psychiatry.

intervention for this population. The After Deployment, Adaptive Parenting Tools (ADAPT) program is a group-based parent training intervention with additional Web-based tools.[62] ADAPT is a 14-week group intervention based on the Parent Management Training Oregon model and has been modified for military families (see **Table 2**, including a review of the 5 positive parenting practices).[63] Adaptations included the importance of reintegrating parents after separation and psychoeducation on how combat stress influences parenting and the family.[62] In an early feasibility study of the first 42 families to receive the intervention, participation rates were high with 79% of families attending at least half of the sessions and 92% attending at least 1. Online learning tools were assessed by the families by 55% at least once and ratings of parent satisfaction were high. Although ADAPT has some similarities with FOCUS in teaching family skills, it is a parent-only–based intervention, whereas FOCUS involves the children directly in the sessions. ADAPT is currently undergoing randomized controlled trials.

STRoNG Military Families and Strong Families Strong Forces

Two similar programs have been designed for use with very young children. The first, STRoNG military families,[64] is designed to work with very young children, aged 0 to 6 years, in National Guard and Reserve families in a 13-session (3 individual family and 10 multifamily group) program. It is designed to improve family functioning through the 5 domains of social support, parenting education, self-care and stress reduction, child routines and parent-child interactions, and care connections for families. It has the potential to provide a model for intervention in families with infants and preschool-aged children. The second intervention, Strong Families Strong Forces, is a home-based reintegration intervention for military families with a recent deployment and a child less than 6 years of age in the home.[65] It teaches parental reflective capacity, developmental relevance, and attachment during postdeployment reintegration. Results from preliminary findings showed a 97% retention rate and increases in parental, self-reflective, and couple reflective capacities as well as improved couple communication and coparenting practices.[66]

Resources

When youth develop moderate to severe mental health symptoms they often need formal treatment services. Community providers who are familiar with military culture and the deployment cycle can provide more effective interventions. Military children seek health care services in the military health community–based network, either when military treatment facilities have limited capacity to treat children or when families live far from military bases. However, these providers often are not trained in military family health and their availability may be limited.[67] Resources have been developed for community providers to assist them in understanding military culture and the unique impact of deployment on families. See **Table 3** for resources, some of which are specifically designed to assist clinicians working with military families; particular attention is given to the Department of Veterans Affairs and Center for Deployment Psychology sites, which offer free online courses for clinicians. Clinicians can offer practical advice and education about coping with deployment for different age groups throughout each stage of deployment (**Table 4**).[2,68]

RESEARCH AND POLICY IMPLICATIONS

Increasing needs for families coping with deployment have led to a significant increase in research surrounding the effects of deployment and military service on children as

Table 4
Family deployment tips

Infants and Toddlers	Preschoolers	School-aged Children	Teenagers
Keep routines predictable	Use simple language to explain the process of deployment	Ask them to help pack deployment bags	May need time to adjust
Use audio/video recordings to stay connected	Make plan to stay connected by sharing treasured item (stuffed animal and send back pictures with the object)	Have a brief goodbye; do not sneak away	May be rebellious, irritable, or more challenging of authority
Be physically and emotionally available to listen	Create a daily ritual to remember the absent parent	Discuss changes in routine but remind them that household rules stay the same	Be alert to high-risk behaviors such as problems with the law, sexual acting out, and drug/alcohol abuse
May need time to warm up on return	Model sharing of emotions; eg, "Mommy is sad because she misses daddy"	Limit TV news watching, watch news with children Be aware of potential dangers; may become irritable, regress, or be fearful of harm to parent	May be distant on return as they continue activities with friends

Data from Osofsky JD, Chartrand MM. Military children from birth to five years. Future Child 2013;23(2):61–77; and AACAP Military Families Resource Center, 2014.

well as development of several interventions. The current research still leaves numerous questions. Military families are often resilient but it is not known how to pace deployment frequency or length to minimize adverse outcomes. Several researchers propose large longitudinal studies to examine these effects.[18,19] Longitudinal studies following military families over time would examine the impacts of military lifestyle, deployments, and sequelae of injury and death of service members for surviving family members. Studying sources of resilience in military family members and the ways to strengthen them may benefit both the development of programs designed to assist military family members and broader populations that face adversity. Public health challenges include disseminating the interventions discussed earlier to providers in wider military and civilian settings. As discussed earlier, families and communities coexist as systems for nurturing healthy growth and development, and distribution of resources to help military-connected children involves clinicians, schools, faith leaders, and other community leaders.

SUMMARY

Families that share a common identity of service, sacrifice, and strength through their contributions to the US military have endured the longest period of sustained service member deployment in 2 generations. Many children have faced these challenges and dealt with the significant impact of prolonged separation from a parent; some families have faced the ultimate sacrifice because of the loss of a service member parent in combat. As shown in this article, research has revealed significant and concerning trends about the repercussions of military deployment on childhood development and behavior. Although there have been limitations to this research caused by the nature of studying a population spread throughout the world, much has been discovered in the past decade that has led to promising interventions and helpful resources for clinicians to assist military families. Although at first glance there is a potential crisis in healthy childhood development and behavior for military-connected children, it is hoped that there is also an opportunity to learn more about the resilience of this population and how the resilience of families facing these challenges can teach clinicians about fostering resilience in all families.

REFERENCES

1. Kelty R, Kleykamp M, Segal DR. The military and the transition to adulthood. Future Child 2010;20(1):181–200.
2. Osofsky JD, Chartrand MM. Military children from birth to five years. Future Child 2013;23(2):61–77
3. Office of the President of the United States. Strengthening our military families: meeting America's commitment. 2011. Available at: http://www.dol.gov/dol/milfamilies/strengthening_our_military_families.pdf. Accessed March 28, 2016.
4. Department of Defense. Demographics profile of the military community. Washington, DC: Office of the Deputy Assistant Secretary of Defense; 2014. Available at: http://download.militaryonesource.mil/12038/MOS/Reports/2014-Demographics-Report.pdf. Accessed March 28, 2016.
5. Hosek J, Wadsworth SM. Economic conditions of military families. Future Child 2013;23(2):41–59.
6. Lundquist JH. Family Formation among women in the U.S. Military: evidence from the NLSY. J Marriage Fam 2005;67:1–13.
7. Franke VC. Generation X and the military: a comparison of attitudes and values between West Point cadets and college students. J Polit Mil Soc 2001;29(1):92–120.
8. Demographics. US Department of Defense education activity. Available at: http://dodea.edu/aboutDoDEA/demographics.cfm. Accessed March 30, 2016.
9. Abb WR. "Citizen Soldier Support Program: CSSP Mapping and Data Center," presentation to the Veterans, Reservists, and Military Families Data and Research Workshop. Washington, September 26, 2012.
10. Clever M, Segal DR. The demographics of military children and families. Future Child 2013;23(2):13–39.
11. Cooney R, Segal MW, DeAngelis K. Moving with the military: race, class, and gender differences in the employment consequences of tied migration. Race, Gender & Class 2011;18(1–2):360–84.
12. Cozza S. Military children and families: introducing the issue. Future Child 2013;23(2):3–11.
13. Gilmore KJ, Meersand P. Normal child and adolescent development: a psychodynamic primer. Arlington (VA): American Psychiatric Publishing; 2014.
14. Glick ID, Berman EM, Clarkin JF, et al. Marital and family therapy. 4th edition. Arlington (VA): American Psychiatric Publishing; 2000.

15. Pincus SH, House R, Christenson J, et al. The emotional cycle of deployment: a military family perspective. US Army Med Dep J 2001;15–23.
16. Bello-Utu CF, DeSocio JE. Military deployment and reintegration: a systematic review of child coping. J Child Adolesc Psychiatr Nurs 2015;28:23–34.
17. Creech SK, Hadley W, Borsari B. The impact of military deployment and reintegration on children and parenting: a systematic review. Prof Psychol Res Pr 2014;45(6):452–64.
18. Lester P, Flake E. How wartime military service affects children and families. Future Child 2013;23(2):121–41.
19. Trautmann J, Alhusen J, Gross D. Impact of deployment on military families with young children: a systematic review. Nurs Outlook 2015;63:656–79.
20. Alfano CA, Lau S, Balderas J, et al. The impact of military deployment on children: placing developmental risk in context. Clin Psychol Rev 2016;43:17–29.
21. Wilson SR, Wilkum K, Chernichky SM, et al. Passport Toward Success: description and evaluation of a program designed to help children and families reconnect after a military deployment. J Appl Commun Res 2011;39(3):223–49.
22. Pfefferbaum B, Houston JB, Sherman MD, et al. Children of National Guard troops deployed in the global war on terrorism. J Loss Trauma 2011;16(4):291–305.
23. Allen ES, Rhoades GK, Stanley SM, et al. On the home front: stress for recently deployed army couples. Fam Process 2011;50(2):235–47.
24. Mansfield AJ, Kaufman JS, Engel CC, et al. Deployment and mental health diagnoses among children of US Army personnel. Arch Pediatr Adolesc Med 2011;165(11):999–1005.
25. Gorman GH, Eide M, Hisle-Gorman E. Wartime military deployment and increased pediatric mental and behavioral health complaints. Pediatrics 2010;126(6):1058–66.
26. Larson MJ, Mohr BA, Adams RS, et al. Association of military deployment of a parent or spouse and changes in dependent use of health care services. Med Care 2012;50(9):821–8.
27. Hisle-Gorman E, Harrington D, Nylund CM, et al. Impact of parents' wartime military deployment and injury on young children's safety and mental health. J Am Acad Child Adolesc Psychiatry 2015;54(4):294–301.
28. Hisle-Gorman E, Eide M, Coll EJ, et al. Attention deficit hyperactivity disorder and medication use by children during parental military deployments. Mil Med 2014;179(5):573–8.
29. Gibbs DA, Martin SL, Kupper LL, et al. Child maltreatment in enlisted soldiers' families during combat-related deployments. JAMA 2007;298(5):528–35.
30. Rabenhorst MM, McCarthy RJ, Thomsen CJ, et al. Child maltreatment among U.S. Air Force parents deployed in support of Operation Iraqi Freedom/Operation Enduring Freedom. Child Maltreat 2015;20(1):61–71.
31. Rentz ED, Marshall SW, Loomis D, et al. Effect of deployment on the occurrence of child maltreatment in military and nonmilitary families. Am J Epidemiol 2007;165(10):1199–206.
32. Engel RC, Gallagher LB, Lyle DS. Military deployments and children's academic achievement: evidence from Department of Defense Education Activity Schools. Econ Educ Rev 2010;29(1):73–82.
33. Richardson A, Chandra A, Martin LT, et al. Effects of soldiers' deployment on children's academic performance and behavioral health. Santa Monica (CA): RAND Corporation; 2011. Available at: http://www.rand.org/content/dam/rand/pubs/monographs/2011/RAND_MG1095.pdf. Accessed March 30, 2016.

34. Tarney CM, Berry-Caban C, Jain RB, et al. Association of spouse deployment on pregnancy outcomes in a U.S. military population. Obstet Gynecol 2015;126(3): 569–74.
35. Levine JA, Bukowinski AT, Sevick CJ, et al. Postpartum depression and timing of spousal military deployment relative to pregnancy and delivery. Arch Gynecol Obstet 2015;292(3):549–58.
36. Nguyen DR, Ee J, Berry-Cabán CS, et al. The effects of military deployment on early child development. US Army Med Dep J 2014;81–6.
37. Barker LH, Berry KD. Developmental issues impacting families with young children during single and multiple deployment. Mil Med 2009;174(10):1033–40.
38. Chartrand MM, Frank DA, White LF, et al. Effect of parents' wartime deployment on the behavior of young children in military families. Arch Pediatr Adolesc Med 2008;162:1009–114.
39. Orthner D, Rose R. Adjustment of army children to deployment separation. Washington, DC: Army Research Institute for the Behavioral and Social Sciences; 2005.
40. Houston JB, Pfefferbaum B, Sherman MD, et al. Children of deployed National Guard troops: perceptions of parental deployment to Operation Iraqi Freedom. Psychiatr Ann 2009;39(8):805–11.
41. Lester P, Peterson K, Reeves J, et al. The long war and parental combat deployment: effects on military children and at-home spouses. J Am Acad Child Adolesc Psychiatry 2010;49(4).310–20.
42. Flake EM, Davis BE, Johnson PL, et al. The psychosocial effects of deployment on military children. J Dev Behav Pediatr 2009;30(4):271–8.
43. Swedean SK, Gonzales MV, Zickefoose BA, et al. Recurrent headache in military-dependent children and the impact of parent deployment. Mil Med 2013;178: 274–8.
44. Chandra A, Lara-Cinisomo S, Jaycox LH, et al. Children on the homefront: the experience of children from military families. Pediatrics 2010;125(1):16–25.
45. Aranda MC, Middleton LS, Flake E, et al. Psychosocial screening in children with wartime-deployed parents. Mil Med 2011;176:402–7.
46. Crow JR, Seybold AK. Discrepancies in military middle-school adolescents' and parents' perceptions of family functioning, social support, anger frequency, and concerns. J Adolesc 2013;36(1):1–9.
47. Barnes VA, Davis H, Treiber FA. Perceived stress, heart rate, and blood pressure among adolescents with family members deployed in Operation Iraqi Freedom. Mil Med 2007;172(1):40–3.
48. Mmari K, Roche KM, Sudhinaraset M, et al. When a parent goes off to war: exploring the issues faced by adolescents and their families. Youth Soc 2009; 40:455–75.
49. Reed SC, Bell JF, Edwards TC. Weapon carrying, physical fighting and gang membership among youth in Washington state military families. Matern Child Health J 2014;18(8):1863–72.
50. Gilreath TD, Cederbaum JA, Astor RA, et al. Substance use among military-connected youth: The California Healthy Kids Survey. Am J Prev Med 2013;44: 150–3.
51. Reed SC, Bell JF, Edwards TC. Adolescent well-being in Washington state military families. Am J Public Health 2011;101:1676–82.
52. Acion L, Ramirez MR, Jorge RE, et al. Increased risk of alcohol and drug use among children from deployed military families. Addiction 2013;108:1418–25.

53. Huebner AJ, Mancini JA. Adjustment among adolescents in military families when a parent is deployed: a final report submitted to the Military Family Research Institute and the Department of Defense Quality of Life Office. Falls Church (VA): Virginia Tech, Department of Human Development; 2005. Available at: http://www.juvenilecouncil.gov/materials/june_8_2007/MFRI%20final%20report%20JUNE%202005.pdf. Accessed March 30, 2016.

54. Chandra A, Lara-Cinisomo S, Jaycox LH, et al. Views from the homefront: the experiences of youth and spouses from military families. Santa Monica (CA): Rand Corporation; 2011. Available at: http://www.rand.org/content/dam/rand/pubs/technical_reports/2011/RAND_TR913.pdf. Accessed March 30, 2016.

55. Chandra A, Burns RM, Tanielian T, et al. Understanding the impact of deployment on children and families. Rand Corporation; 2008. Available at: http://www.rand.org/content/dam/rand/pubs/working_papers/2008/RAND_WR566.pdf. Accessed March, 30, 2016.

56. O'Connell ME, Boat T, Warner KE. Preventing mental, emotional, and behavioral disorders among young people: progress and possibilities. Washington, DC: National Academies Press; 2009.

57. Lester P, Liang LJ, Milburn N, et al. Evaluation of a family-centered preventive intervention for military families: parent and child longitudinal outcomes. J Am Acad Child Adolesc Psychiatry 2016;55(1):14–24.

58. Rotheram-Borus MJ, Lee M, Lin YY, et al. Six-year intervention outcomes for adolescent children of parents with the human immunodeficiency virus. Arch Pediatr Adolesc Med 2004;158(8):742–8.

59. Beardslee WR, Wright EJ, Gladstone TR, et al. Long-term effects from a randomized trial of two public health preventive interventions for parental depression. J Fam Psychol 2007;21(4):703.

60. Layne CM, Saltzman WR, Poppleton L, et al. Effectiveness of a school-based group psychotherapy program for war-exposed adolescents: a randomized controlled trial. J Am Acad Child Adolesc Psychiatry 2008;47(9):1048–62.

61. Beardslee W, Lester P, Klosinski L, et al. Family-centered preventive intervention for military families: implications for implementation science. Prev Sci 2011;12(4):339–48.

62. Gewirtz AH, Pinna KL, Hanson SK, et al. Promoting parenting to support reintegrating military families: after deployment, adaptive parenting tools. Psychol Serv 2014;11(1):31.

63. Forgatch MS, Patterson GR. Parent Management Training—Oregon Model: an intervention for antisocial behavior in children and adolescents. In: Weisz JR, Kazdin AE, editors. Evidence-based psychotherapies for children and adolescents. 2nd edition. New York: Guilford Press; 2010. p. 159–78.

64. Rosenblum KL, Muzik M. STRoNG intervention for military families with young children. Psychiatr Serv 2014;65:399.

65. DeVoe ER, Ross AM, Paris R. Build it together and they will come: the case for community-based participatory research with military populations. Adv Soc Work 2012;13(1):149–65.

66. DeVoe E, Ross AM. Engaging and retaining National Guard/Reserve families with very young children in treatment: The Strong Families Strong Forces Program. CYF News 2013. Available at: http://www.apa.org/pi/families/resources/newsletter/2013/01/strong-families.aspx.

67. American Psychological Association (APA) Presidential Task Force on Military Deployment Services for Youth, Families and Service Members. The psychological needs of US military service members and their families: A preliminary

report. 2007. Available at: http://www.apa.org/about/policy/military-deployment-services/pdf. Accessed April 1, 2016.

68. American Academy of Child and Adolescent Psychiatry (AACAP) Military Families Resource Center. 2014. Available at: http://www.aacap.org/AACAP/Families_and_Youth/Resource_Centers/Military_Families_Resource_Center/Home.aspx. Accessed April 1, 2016.

Growing up – or not – with Gun Violence

Judy Schaechter, MD, MBA*, Patricia G. Alvarez, MD

KEYWORDS

• Firearms • Injuries • Child development • Counseling • Safe storage • Violence

KEY POINTS

• Firearm violence can disrupt normal child development.
• In combination with normal child developmental stages, firearms pose significant risk of death, injury, and psychosocial trauma.
• Speaking to children is not enough to prevent firearm violence.
• Prevention of firearm violence requires adult responsibility, including methods to reduce child/adolescent access to firearms.

INTRODUCTION

Death is the ultimate interference with child development. Firearm violence has the potential to disrupt child development completely, by causing premature child death, or to hinder normal health via the loss of family members, guilt from having pulled the trigger (unintentional or otherwise), stress of chronic community violence, the ominous threat of mass shootings, or even accumulated adverse responses to media violence. Unintentional injury is the leading cause of death in children and adults aged 1 to 44 years and the fourth most common cause of death in the overall population.[1] Gun trauma may cause physical, emotional, and mental health disruption to injured victims as well as to those who were not directly in a bullet's trajectory.

Firearm injury prevention research has been insufficiently funded for decades.[2] Children have been among the victims of mass shootings and have experienced the consequences of interpersonal, family, and community violence that occurs in homes and streets on a daily basis.[3] Studies have enumerated pediatric firearm death and injury; additional research catalogues the consequences of violent trauma to children and adolescents,[4] including physical and behavioral disruptions, assault recidivism, perpetration of violence, and negative socioeconomic outcomes.[5,6] Research-based guidance

Disclosure: The authors have no relevant disclosures.
Department of Pediatrics, University of Miami Miller School of Medicine and Holtz Children's Hospital at Jackson Health Systems, 1601 Northwest 12th Avenue, Miami, FL 33136, USA
* Corresponding author.
E-mail address: JSchaech@med.miami.edu

pediatric.theclinics.com

about how to prevent firearm violence caused by or inflicted on children and adolescents provides insight, but no clear map toward elimination.[7] More questions remain than answers. There is still more to discover about the interplay between normal child and adolescent growth, mental health, learning, attention and firearm access, ownership, handling, play, shooting, and violence. In addition, risk and outcome variances that might be caused by differences posed by conditions of mental illness, chronic disease, learning or attention disorders, and social determinants either in children or their household members and how these affect firearm injury risk or should inform policy have not been completely described.

Despite seemingly daily headlines, the consequences of gun injury on children's lives and development and, relatedly, how child growth and development influence gun events are incompletely understood. However, where associations are strong, such as accumulated research indicating a direct relationship between firearm availability and risk of homicide, suicide, and unintentional gun injury, there is less science on how to meaningfully reduce that availability, at least in the United States.[8,9] This omission is of great concern, because firearm injury accounts for nearly 18% of all deaths in the United States; almost as many deaths as those caused by car crashes.[10] Unlike motor vehicle deaths, the number of firearm deaths has not decreased over the past half-decade, but instead its slight increase has been driven largely by suicides.[9]

GUN INJURIES

Gun injuries are a leading cause of death for children and adolescents.[11] The United States outpaces all other high-income countries in overall firearm death, firearm homicide, firearm suicide, and unintentional firearm deaths by several-fold.[12] Most homicides and suicides in the United States are firearm homicides and suicides. The more guns there are, the higher the burden of violence: for every 1% increase in household gun ownership, youth firearm homicide increases 2.4%.[13]

Firearm suicide accounts for approximately two-thirds of all US firearm deaths, although firearm homicide outnumbers firearm suicides among the young. Unintentional deaths are harder to accurately enumerate, because such incidents, particularly among children, may be coded as homicides or suicides in vital statistics data.[14,15]

However, even when such data are used, unintentional firearm death disproportionately affects youth.[16] In 2014, 106 children died of unintentional firearm-related injuries.[17] Unintentional firearm injuries are among the top 10 leading causes of injury-related deaths for children aged 7 to 16 years.[17] These shootings occur most often when children gain access to an unsecured firearm in a home.[11,18,19]

Pediatric firearm homicide may also occur close to home. When the source of the gun is known, it often did not come further than friends and family. Most school shooters obtained their guns from home or a relative.[20] The origin of guns used by youth in crimes is more storied. A national sample of incarcerated youth who committed crimes as juveniles reported that 47% of their guns came from the street or black market, whereas 38% were obtained from a friend or family member.[21]

NORMAL CHILD DEVELOPMENT AND RISK OF FIREARM INJURY

Pediatrics is concerned with optimal child growth, development, and health. Pediatricians follow patients from birth into adulthood and ensure their continued development, often assessing progress against recognizable milestones. As children journey through development, they interact with their environment. Their growth stage poses challenges and even risks that differ based on physical, emotional, and cognitive abilities. In every developmental phase, child and adolescent curiosity, which propels those reaching for maturity to explore, puts them in contact with new objects, situations, and contexts, often in ways their prior developmental stage did not prepare them to encounter. A child's ever-increasing independence and changing developmental tasks require that they learn, and potentially confront risk, in new ways, within varying contexts. As children progress, parents may not always understand a child's full developmental capacities or the limits of those capacities, which operate within normal ranges rather than fixed points, and fluctuate over time even within the same child.

Early Childhood/Preschool

Thus, once fully dependent newborns surprise parents when they roll off a bed or first learn to scoot and fall down a step. The physical capacity and evolving independence of toddlers surely contributes to the unexpected shootings by this age group.[22] Toddlers are developmentally able to find firearms left in purses, drawers, on shelves, or under bedding. The combination of new physical skills and strengths, the need to interact with the environment, but also an inability to recognize or even cognitively conceive of an object's potential lethality places very young children in harm's way when there is access to loaded firearms. For the very young, the world is to be experienced without fear of harm. Toddlers are supposed to touch and pick up everything they find, and even put such things in their mouths. Slightly older children still see such objects as toys or other irresistible items of curiosity, and this is normal. Even if an adult speaks with a child of such an age, imploring the child to restrain from a certain behavior, impulse control has not developed in preschoolers.[23] Thus, it is predictable that children 2, 3, and even 4 years of age will shoot themselves or someone else when they find a loaded firearm in a bedroom, car, or another unsecured location.[24–26]

School Age

Parents speak with their older, school-aged children about concepts such as danger causing pain, and what not to touch, but, developmentally, school-aged children should not be depended on to never touch things that might be dangerous, or to always follow a parent's instructions, especially when the parent is not present. Developmental gains are incomplete and lapses occur regularly. Conceptualization of finality, which is required to fully understand death, does not usually begin until approximately age 7 years. Understanding causality begins in early childhood, but continues to develop through adolescence. Grasping the concept of the action of handling a gun and the lethal consequence of injury or death is still abstract for many children, particularly when they see so many images of guns in the media, often displayed with little to no consequence for their heroes. For school-aged children, firearm injury, by all intents, ranks as the fourth leading cause of injury death.[17] By age 11 years, firearm injury is the second leading cause of injury death.[27] Children in this age group increasingly seek independence, but are also subject to peer pressure, which may encourage them to investigate firearm mechanisms, power, and potential, even when that contradicts parental advice.

Early Adolescence

Advancing elementary and middle school youth are often anxious to imitate older teens and adults, but may also rebel as they realize parents are not perfect. Although they understand right from wrong, it is normal at this stage for young adolescents to test rules and push limits, and to question authority. Their expressive skills are not yet fully developed and so they may put feelings into action rather than words, sometimes leading to physical conflict or self-harm.

Adolescents' emotional growth is not necessarily linear; they may revert to more immature behaviors, particularly under stress.[28] Under such conditions, access to weapons presents risk. A study of more than 6000 fifth to seventh graders in the nonmetropolitan southeast, reported that 46% themselves owned guns (including BB/pellet guns). Nearly a quarter reported owning firearms (rifles, shotguns, pistols, or handguns). These firearms were in addition to family guns, reported by more than 70% of the students. Of concern, but predictable and consistent with young adolescent development, 11.3% of the adolescent gun owners reported using the gun to frighten someone and 5.5% had brought it to school at least once.[29]

Advancing Adolescence

Even older adolescence presents developmental challenges. Cognitively, much growth has occurred, but emotional regulation is incomplete. The executive functions, required for impulse control, are among the last to mature, and do not do so at the same rate among all youth. However, there are too many examples in every community of adolescents who hastily claimed their own lives, who acted recklessly and harmed another, who were not intending any harm but were nonetheless playing with a gun that went off. Sometimes teens really were in the wrong place at the wrong time; in other cases, they made an impulsive decision or a regrettable safety omission because they were behaving as teenagers.[30] In every case, both the tissue damage and the emotional trauma are serious. Adolescence is a time to be protected from gun violence, not to be experimenting with it.

Weapon carrying may occur with less frequency among urban teens than rural teens, who are more accustomed to the hunting and sporting culture. Nonetheless, youth firearm carrying occurs throughout the United States. Per the Youth Risk Behavior Surveillance Survey, in 2013, 5.5% of high schoolers carried guns in the 30 days before the survey.[31]

An adolescent propensity for violence, at least on the part of some teens, though most often temporary, should not be ignored. Violence victimization and perpetration, both in general and specifically with firearms, increases during adolescence into the early adult years. Adolescents are more likely to be victims of bullying, assault, and violent crime than other age cohorts. Being a victim of violence puts people at risk for violence perpetration. A compelling study regarding the cycle of violence found that exposure to firearm violence doubled the probability that an adolescent would perpetrate serious violence within 2 years.[32] The good news is that, for the greatest proportion of teens, the adolescent spike in experienced violence decreases.[33] The decrease in aggression and assault perpetration coincides with adolescent maturation, particularly developmental gains in impulsiveness and self-control. The adolescent/young adult period is a time of particular developmental risk regarding firearm violence. Protecting adolescents from firearm violence, both as victims and perpetrators, while their own development matures may be key to individual and community health.

FIREARM INJURY, VIOLENCE, BEHAVIOR, AND MENTAL HEALTH

The lifetime prevalence of mental illness approaches half the overall population. The most common of these conditions, anxiety, mood, and behavioral disorders, begin during childhood and adolescence. Substance use also often has its origins during adolescence. Prevalence of such disorders during childhood and adolescence approximates 22%.[34]

Per the Youth Risk Behavior Surveillance Survey, 29.9% of high school students nationwide had felt so sad or hopeless almost every day for 2 or more consecutive weeks that they stopped doing some usual activities, 13.6% of students had made a plan to attempt suicide, and 8% had attempted suicide during the past 12 months.[35] According to the National Health and Nutrition Examination Survey, 7.8% of children 3 to 17 years old had learning disorders; 7.9% had attention-deficit/hyperactivity disorder; and 5.9% had autism, intellectual delays, or other developmental delays.[36] Many of these conditions place affected youth at higher risk of self-inflicted and impulsive firearm injury. An accessible firearm is one of the most concerning risk factors for suicidal patients.[37]

The risk of violent acts committed against others is nominally higher among those with severe mental illness than among the general population.[38] Although mental illness is often thought to contribute significantly to assault violence, only 3% to 5% of such violence in the United States might be so attributed.[39] Signs that someone may commit violence are the same among the severely mentally ill as in the population overall.[40] More than mental illness per se, low self-control, which corresponds with higher impulsivity, has been found to be among the strongest correlates of crime, delinquency, violence, and other problem behaviors.[33]

MENTAL HEALTH CONSEQUENCES OF VICTIMIZATION

Further research defining the relationships between pediatric firearm violence, behavior, and mental health is still much needed. Injury and violence generally can increase the risk of morbidities such as posttraumatic stress disorder, mood disorders, and substance abuse. These same conditions may predate violence and potentially increase a person's risk of disturbance after a violent event. However, how such factors interact with each other; individual, family, and community contexts; and what tools can meaningfully predict or prevent further assault victimization, self-harm, or perpetration of violence against others is less clear.

CHILD SHOOTERS

In the case of unintentional firearm shooting by a child, the traumatic consequences of survivor's guilt may be significant. As a 10-year-old child, Sean Smith found his father's unlocked and loaded gun when he was looking for video games. Pulling the trigger, he mistakenly shot his 8-year-old sister when she ran by. She died in his lap while Sean called 911. Now a recovering adult, Sean attributes his drug use, school dropout, and other behavioral problems as a teen and younger adult to the pain that followed him after the shooting.[41] There is little research on child shooter survivors, their outcomes, or how to treat them. The best means to prevent their trauma seems to be empirically obvious: to reduce or eliminate child and adolescent access to firearms and ammunition.

COMMUNITY VIOLENCE

High exposure to community violence tends to occur in communities with low social capital, high levels of poverty, and high crime. Families in these communities experience multiple sources of stress, which may include unstable housing, reduced opportunities for youth, high levels of school dropout, unemployment, incarceration, and other factors known to put children at risk.

Children 7 to 12 years old exposed to high rates of community violence tended to show more externalizing behaviors, showed impaired social and behavioral functioning, and were more likely to come from families with high levels of conflict and low cohesiveness.[42] Early studies of children exposed to high levels of chronic community violence revealed similar findings, and association with high-risk behaviors, including fighting and gun and knife carrying.[43] Exposure to community violence seems to increase aggressive behaviors, not only in the near term but also long term, through changes in social cognition.[44] Community violence exposure was related to increases in aggressive behavior and depression among fifth and seventh graders, which persists a year later, and was observed even after controlling for prior affective issues, family functioning, and parenting style.[45]

COMMUNITY VIOLENCE, VICTIMIZATION, AND WEAPON CARRYING

Violence experienced by children leads to negative outcomes and is a public health concern.[46–49] A recent systematic review of the literature determined that approximately 1 billion children worldwide experienced violence in the past year.[46] This exposure to violence has led some researchers to develop models for youth weapon carrying:

- The drug-gun diffusion model of youth carrying describes youth who carry for self-defense in response to violence in the area.[47,50]
- The stepping-stone model describes how previous episodes of violence prime the desire to carry for the future.[47]
- The cumulative-risk model of youth gun carrying takes into consideration all the risk factors that lead to weapon carrying: both participation in violence and exposure to violence.[47]

There are several risk factors for weapon carrying, including gender, gang participation, drug and alcohol use, lack of adult support, poor academic performance, witnessing violence and victimization, lack of safe play spaces, and history of aggression.[50–53] Risk subsets can be stratified, even across high-risk areas. A Chicago study found that 4.9% of boys aged 9 to 19 years had carried a firearm.[53] However, a study in Flint, Michigan, of assault-injured youth visiting an emergency room revealed that 23% of patients had reported possession of a firearm within the past 6 months.[54]

Programs seeking to reduce weapon carrying have been designed to address overall well-being, build adult mentorship programs, and provide alternatives to gang involvement.[52] However, at least 1 survey shows that students from low-income neighborhoods stated they felt safer when they had a gun or other weapon to protect themselves.[55]

GUN SAFETY PROGRAMS, PARENT PERCEPTIONS, AND TOYS AS FUNCTIONS OF CHILD DEVELOPMENT

Given the potentially lethal risks loaded firearms pose when accessible to children, programs have been developed to educate children on gun violence and safety. However, there is no evidence that such programs are effective in reducing injury or even keeping children from avoiding gun play. Perhaps the best known program is the National Rifle Association's Eddie Eagle GunSafe Program. Initially launched in 1988 and updated in 2015, it is designed for children from prekindergarten to fourth grade. The basic avoidance message is "Stop! Don't touch. Run away. Tell a grown-up."[56] There is no research evidence that it is effective with children. Another gun safety program, STAR (Straight Talk About Risks), was developed by the Center to Prevent Handgun Violence to target children in prekindergarten through 12th grade. It also adopted a "Just say no" approach, adding lessons about good decision making, peer pressure, emotions that lead to violence, and consequences of gun violence.[57] However, STAR was evaluated by an independent research team. Children 4 to 7 years of age who went through the STAR program and controls were observed in a structured play area filled with toys, plus a toy gun and a real gun. There was no difference in the likelihood of playing with the firearm once found. The researchers concluded that "Stop! Don't Touch!" approaches for children do not keep them safe.[57]

Many parents do not fully know of or believe this evidence. Parents tend to trust that their children know better. A random digit dial survey found that 87% of parents of children 5 to 15 years of age said their children would not touch a gun under any circumstances if they found one. More than half said their children were too smart or knew better than to handle a gun if they found one. Only 12% of the gun owners reported that they stored their guns locked and unloaded, revealing that more gun owners were relying on their children to stay away from the guns than their own active protections, such as the use of gun locks or safes. Even for the younger children (5–9 years old), 85% of parents said their children would act responsibly. Eighty-nine percent of parents of children aged 10 to 14 years and 93% of parents of 15-year-olds concurred that their children would not touch a found gun.[58]

However, in terms of normal child development, these expectations may be unrealistic for school-aged and teenaged children who do not reliably weigh consequences, avoid temptation, resist peer pressure, and have fully developed executive function.

An experiment was designed in which boys 8 to 12 years old were observed through a 2-way mirror. Parents were invited to watch behind the mirror. On the other side of the mirror, children entered an examination room. Hidden within the examination room were water guns and an unloaded real gun. Three-fourths of parents thought their sons would not touch the real gun if found. Within 15 minutes 76% of the boys found and handled the real gun. Half reported that they thought it was a toy or were not sure. Half of those who handled the real gun pulled the trigger hard enough to fire the gun. More than 90% of the children who handled the gun said they had previously received gun safety instructions, some from an instructor or police.[59]

In a study of 314 parent-child pairs, 64% of parents reported keeping firearms in their homes. A substantial proportion (39%) of parents reported that their children did not know the location of the gun in the home, and yet their children reported that they did know where the guns were stored. Nearly a quarter of parents who said their children had never touched a household gun were contradicted by their children. Children less than 10 years of age were as likely as older children to know where the household gun was located (75%) and to report having handled the gun (36%).[60]

Despite such findings, a sizable number of parents trust very young children even with loaded guns. Nearly a quarter of gun-owning parents reported that they would trust their 4-year-old to 12-year-old children with a loaded firearm.[61] Another study reported that 14% of gun owners would trust children less than 12 years old with loaded firearms, and most reported that they would trust children by age 13 years.[62]

Although some parents think they can trust their children with loaded firearms, they may be missing key developmental information, including that many children keep information to themselves, and that it can be developmentally normal to keep secrets. Not all children share with parents a full account of their activities; they may particularly withhold information of which they believe their parents would not approve.

A survey of California youth 12 to 18 years old revealed that 5% admitted to handling guns without their parents' knowledge. This handling is usually a social activity, because 69% of the time it was with friends, it was often for fun, and frequently involved shooting the gun (49%). Nearly half of the guns used came from the teen's own home or that of a friend or relative.[63]

Parents' potential overestimate of a child's developmental abilities can lead to other risky conclusions regarding firearm access. Forty-six percent of gun-owning parents reported believing that children 0 to 6 years of age could tell the difference between a real and a toy gun (although only 10% of nonowning parents thought the same).[62] This belief is likely a significant and dangerous overestimate of young children's ability, as pointed out by both the Jackman and colleagues[59] and Hardy studies.[57] Further, such parents are likely unaware of how much imitation guns may resemble genuine firearms, and likewise, in the era of plastic guns that are absolutely authentic, how much real firearms resemble toys. The Ninth Circuit Court of Appeals reasoned that a plastic toy gun may be indistinguishable from a real gun in appearance, and that case involved adults as observers, including a gun owner with prior military experience.[64] The best-trained adult personnel are often confused, to unfortunate or even tragic ends. In many cases, there is little or nothing to visibly distinguish a toy gun from a real gun, as law enforcement personnel have reported. Children have been fatally shot by police officers who thought the youth were brandishing real guns.[65] A National Institute of Justice Study replicating various scenarios with real and toy guns revealed that, depending on the look of the toy gun, as many as 96% of officers shot at an assailant with a toy gun (marked with an orange tip) when confronted in a simulation.[66]

In a separate study by the Bureau of Justice, 458 police departments were asked about toy guns involved in law enforcement encounters over 4-year period. Imitation guns were used in 15% of robberies (5654) and 8128 assaults. There were 1128 events in which law enforcement threatened to use force because an officer thought an imitation gun was real, and in 252 incidents force was used because an officer thought the replica gun was real. The departments surveyed seized 31,650 imitation guns.[67]

The difficulty distinguishing between real and toy guns extends to the Transportation Safety Administration as well, as was evident when a young boy's toy gun resulted in the 2-hour shutdown of Charlotte-Douglas International Airport, the evacuation of 4 concourses, and the delaying of 50 airplanes over the Thanksgiving holiday in 2000.[68]

If adults, and even those trained in firearms, do not readily distinguish toy guns from real guns, then parents should not anticipate that their children can do so. This ability seems to be not only a developmental issue but also a functional/mechanical issue related to the approximation many imitation guns have to their genuine counterparts, and vice versa. It has also been suggested that the full scope of the dangers of toy guns, how they should be regulated, and how regulations should be enforced has not been resolved or even adequately studied.[65,69]

PREVENTION

Promotion of healthy child development means mitigation of violence; reduction of firearm injury risk; and attention to the strengths and vulnerabilities of families, schools, and communities and the supports around them.

Teaching children to avoid guns is not enough, because it does not work and is not developmentally appropriate. The onus of prevention for firearm access leading to injury and other consequences is on adults, the guardians of the children, the community, and the legal owners of the firearms.

PROPER STORAGE: LIMIT ACCESS FOR CHILDREN'S SAKE

Consistent with the policy of The American Academy of Pediatrics, children are safest in environments without firearms.[70] That approach is the least risky. However, guns are ubiquitous in the United States. More than 30% of homes have firearms.[71] Gun owners, including extended family and friends, should be certain that all firearms are stored unloaded and locked, which means that firearms are not just out of sight, hidden up high, in a drawer or under a seat in the car. Parents need to secure their own homes and then ask about the places where they and their children visit.

FIREARM ACCESS AND PREVENTION: CHILD ACCESS PREVENTION LAWS

Child access prevention (CAP) laws have been established with the expectation that adult gun owners will safely store firearms, because these laws make owners criminally liable if children gain access to a firearm and injures themselves or others.[72–75] More than 17 states have enacted CAP laws. The effects of these laws have been inconsistent across states. States that implemented early and as a felony seem to be most effective at reducing unintentional firearm injury.

PHYSICIAN COUNSELING

Parents may not understand all of child development and its impact concerning the risk of firearm violence, so pediatricians and other child health clinicians can work with them to help clarify normal child behavior, in an effort to mitigate risk and potentiate adult protection of child safety.

There is evidence that physician counseling regarding safe storage is effective. In a randomized controlled study of parents of children 2 to 11 years old, pediatricians recommended safe storage, resulting in a 21.4% increase in the use of gun locks.[76] Another study evaluating single sessions by a clinician found some increase in those who purchased a trigger lock.[77] A study of parents revealed that 90%, gun owners or not, would be willing to tell their pediatricians whether they kept a gun in the home. Nearly all said they would follow their pediatrician's advice about gun storage.[62]

SUMMARY

Pediatricians must remember that they not only care for children but also their parents. Most parents who own firearms see their weapons as means to protect their children. Because of this, clinicians need to approach the topic in a nonadversarial way and work together with the family to develop a plan for keeping their children safe. The issue should continue to be addressed at an individual level during well-child visits by providing a supportive place for parents, family members, and physicians to discuss effective, safe ways of storing firearms. Pediatricians could also address the issue at a community level by engaging the neighborhoods where children live and play and by working with city planners and police departments in order to provide safe outdoor spaces.

Unless there is significant interference, most children will grow, develop along a normal trajectory, and thrive. For some children, deadly interference comes in the form of a single bullet delivered through the barrel of an unsecured gun, left by an unsuspecting gun owner, most likely someone known to the child victim. For others, significant interference comes as a constellation of factors, some individual (eg, depression, anxiety, or delayed executive function), along with family and community factors (eg, adverse childhood events, poverty, high crime rate, neighborhood stress, and suboptimal schooling). It is the job of pediatricians, educators, law enforcement, parents, child advocates, and gun owners to keep children and adolescents safe. That means being aware of how vulnerable children are as they grow toward adulthood and how their behavior and capabilities change according to their development. More than anything, it should be recognized that keeping weapons and children separated is an adult responsibility.

REFERENCES

1. CDC WISQARS 10 leading causes of death by age group, United States - 2013. Available at: http://www.cdc.gov/injury/images/lc-charts/leading_causes_of_death_by_age_group_2013-a.gif. Accessed February 8, 2016.
2. Kellermann AL, Rivara FP. Silencing the science on gun research. JAMA 2013; 309(6):549–50.
3. Groves B, Zuckerman B, Marans S, et al. Silent victims. Children who witness violence. JAMA 1993;269(2):262–4.
4. Pine DS, Cohen JA. Trauma in children and adolescents: risk and treatment of psychiatric sequelae. Biol Psychiatry 2002;51(7):519–31.
5. Cunningham RM, Carter PM, Ranney M, et al. Violent reinjury and mortality among youth seeking emergency department care for assault-related injury: a 2-year prospective cohort study. JAMA Pediatr 2015;169(1):63–70.
6. Greenspan AI, Kellermann AL. Physical and psychological outcomes 8 months after serious gunshot injury. J Trauma 2002;53(4):709–16.
7. Hardy MS. Behavior-oriented approaches to reducing youth gun violence. Future Child 2002;12(2):100–17.
8. Hemenway D. Private guns, public health. United States of America. Ann Arbor, MI: The University of Michigan Press; 2004.
9. Steinbrook R, Stern RJ, Redberg RF. Firearm injuries and gun violence: call for papers. JAMA Intern Med 2016;176(5):596–7.
10. Xu J, Kochanek KD, Bastian BA. National vital statistics reports. Available at: http://www.cdc.gov/nchs/data/nvsr/nvsr64/nvsr64_02.pdf. Accessed April 16, 2016.
11. Faulkenberry JG, Schaechter J. Reporting on pediatric unintentional firearm injury–who's responsible. J Trauma Acute Care Surg 2015;79(3 Suppl 1):S2–8.
12. Richardson EG, Hemenway D. Homicide, suicide, and unintentional firearm fatality: comparing the United States with other high-income countries, 2003. J Trauma 2011;70(1):238–43.
13. Miller M, Hemenway D, Azrael D. State-level homicide victimization rates in the US in relation to survey measures of household firearm ownership, 2001-2003. Soc Sci Med 2007;64(3):656–64.
14. Barber C, Hemenway D. Too many or too few unintentional firearm deaths in official U.S. mortality data? Accid Anal Prev 2011;43(3):724–31.
15. Schaechter J, Duran I, De Marchena J, et al. Are "accidental" gun deaths as rare as they seem? A comparison of medical examiner manner of death coding with an intent-based classification approach. Pediatrics 2003;111(4 Pt 1):741–4.
16. Karch DL, Logan J, McDaniel D, et al. Surveillance for violent deaths–National Violent Death Reporting System, 16 states, 2009. MMWR Surveill Summ 2012; 61(6):1–43.
17. US Centers for Disease Control and Prevention (CDC). National Center for Injury Prevention and Control. Available at: http://www.cdc.gov/injury/wisqars. Accessed April 19, 2016.
18. Coyne-Beasley T, Schoenbach VJ, Johnson RM. "Love our kids, lock your guns": a community-based firearm safety counseling and gun lock distribution program. Arch Pediatr Adolesc Med 2001;155(6):659–64.

19. Hemenway D, Barber C, Miller M. Unintentional firearm deaths: a comparison of other-inflicted and self-inflicted shootings. Accid Anal Prev 2010;42(4):1184–8.

20. Vossekuil B. The final report and findings of the Safe School Initiative: implications for the prevention of school attacks in the United States. Lollingdale, PA: DIANE Publishing; 2002.

21. Webster DW, Freed LH, Frattaroli S, et al. How delinquent youths acquire guns: initial versus most recent gun acquisitions. J Urban Health 2002;79(1):60–9.

22. Ingraham C. People are getting shot by toddlers on a weekly basis this year. The Washington Post. 2015. Available at: https://www.washingtonpost.com/news/wonk/wp/2015/10/14/people-are-getting-shot-by-toddlers-on-a-weekly-basis-this-year/. Accessed April 14, 2016.

23. Evans AD, Lee K. Emergence of lying in very young children. Dev Psychol 2013; 49(10):1958–63.

24. Schramm R, Harris R. 3-year-old shoots self in face; mother arrested. 2014. Available at: http://www.cbs46.com/story/26286195/3-year-old-shot-in-nw-atlanta. Accessed January 28, 2016.

25. Martinez M, Marco T. Mom fatally shot when son, 2, grabs fun from her purse in Walmart. 2014. Available at: http://www.cnn.com/2014/12/30/us/idaho-walmart-shooting-accident-mother-toddler/. Accessed January 28, 2016.

26. WCBD News. 4-year-old SC boy shoots himself while at grandparents house. 2014. Available at: http://wbtw.com/2014/05/13/4-year-old-sc-boy-shoots-himself-while-at-grandparents-house/. Accessed January 28, 2016.

27. Nance ML, Krummel TM, Oldham KT, et al. Firearm injuries and children: a policy statement of the American Pediatric Surgical Association. J Am Coll Surg 2013; 217(5):940–6.

28. Spano S. ACT for Youth Upstate Center for Excellence. Research fACTs and findings. Available at: http://www.actforyouth.net/resources/rf/rf_stages_0504.pdf. Accessed April 16, 2016.

29. Cunningham PB, Henggeler SW, Limber SP, et al. Patterns and correlates of gun ownership among nonmetropolitan and rural middle school students. J Clin Child Psychol 2000;29(3):432–42.

30. Rich JA. Wrong place, wrong time: trauma and violence in the lives of young black men. Baltimore, MD: JHU Press; 2009.

31. Centers for Disease Control and Prevention (CDC). Youth Risk Behavior Surveillance System - United States, 2013. MMWR Suppl 2014;63(4):1–168.

32. Bingenheimer JB, Brennan RT, Earls FJ. Firearm violence exposure and serious violent behavior. Science 2005;308(5726):1323–6.

33. Loeber R, Farrington DP. From juvenile delinquency to adult crime: criminal careers, justice policy and prevention. Oxford: Oxford University Press; 2012.

34. Kessler RC, Berglund P, Demler O, et al. Lifetime prevalence and age-of-onset distributions of DSM-IV disorders in the National Comorbidity Survey Replication. Arch Gen Psychiatry 2005;62(6):593–602.

35. Centers for Disease Control and Prevention (CDC). Morbidity and mortality weekly report. Available at: http://www.cdc.gov/mmwr/pdf/ss/ss6304.pdf. Accessed April 16, 2016.

36. Schieve LA, Gonzalez V, Boulet SL, et al. Concurrent medical conditions and health care use and needs among children with learning and behavioral developmental disabilities, National Health Interview Survey, 2006-2010. Res Dev Disabil 2012;33(2):467–76.

37. Miller M, Barber C, White RA, et al. Firearms and suicide in the United States: is risk independent of underlying suicidal behavior? Am J Epidemiol 2013;178(6): 946–55.

38. Appelbaum PS. Public safety, mental disorders, and guns. JAMA Psychiatry 2013;70(6):565–6.

39. Swanson JW. Mental disorder, substance abuse, and community violence: an epidemiological approach. Violence and mental disorder: developments in risk assessment. Chicago: The University of Chicago Press; 1994. p. 101–36.

40. Van Dorn R, Volavka J, Johnson N. Mental disorder and violence: is there a relationship beyond substance use? Soc Psychiatry Psychiatr Epidemiol 2012;47(3): 487–503.

41. Kids and guns: coping with an accidental shooting [video]. Available at. http://www.cnn.com/videos/tv/2015/10/22/kids-and-guns-kaye-dnt-ac.cnn/video/playlists/guns-in-america/. Accessed February 8, 2016.

42. Cooley-Quille MR, Turner SM, Beidel DC. Emotional impact of children's exposure to community violence: a preliminary study. J Am Acad Child Adolesc Psychiatry 1995;34(10):1362–8.

43. Huesmann LR, Guerra NG. Children's normative beliefs about aggression and aggressive behavior. J Pers Soc Psychol 1997;72(2):408–19.

44. Guerra NG, Huesmann LR, Spindler A. Community violence exposure, social cognition, and aggression among urban elementary school children. Child Dev 2003;74(5):1561–76.

45. Gorman-Smith D, Tolan P. The role of exposure to community violence and developmental problems among inner-city youth. Dev Psychopathol 1998;10(1): 101–16.

46. Hillis S, Mercy J, Amobi A, et al. Global prevalence of past-year violence against children: a systematic review and minimum estimates. Pediatrics 2016;30(24): 2038–50.

47. Spano R, Pridemore WA, Bolland J. Specifying the role of exposure to violence and violent behavior on initiation of gun carrying: a longitudinal test of three models of youth gun carrying. J Interpers Violence 2012;27(1):158–76.

48. Leeb RT, Barker LE, Strine TW. The effect of childhood physical and sexual abuse on adolescent weapon carrying. J Adolesc Health 2007;40(6):551–8.

49. Pabayo R, Molnar BE, Kawachi I. The role of neighborhood income inequality in adolescent aggression and violence. J Adolesc Health 2014;55(4):571–9.

50. Vaughn MG, Perron BE, Abdon A, et al. Correlates of handgun carrying among adolescents in the United States. J Interpers Violence 2012;27(10):2003–21.

51. Carter PM, Walton MA, Roehler DR, et al. Firearm violence among high-risk emergency department youth after an assault injury. Pediatrics 2015;135(5):805–15.

52. Hemenway D, Vriniotis M, Johnson RM, et al. Gun carrying by high school students in Boston, MA: does overestimation of peer gun carrying matter? J Adolesc 2011;34(5):997–1003.

53. Molnar BE, Miller MJ, Azrael D, et al. Neighborhood predictors of concealed firearm carrying among children and adolescents: results from the project on human development in Chicago neighborhoods. Arch Pediatr Adolesc Med 2004; 158(7):657–64.

54. Carter PM, Walton MA, Newton MF, et al. Firearm possession among adolescents presenting to an urban emergency department for assault. Pediatrics 2013; 132(2):213–21.

55. Vacha EF, McLaughlin TF. Risky firearms behavior in low-income families of elementary school children: the impact of poverty, fear of crime, and crime victimization on keeping and storing firearms. J Fam Violence 2004;19(3):175–84.
56. Eddie Eagle Gunsafe Program. Available at: https://eddieeagle.nra.org/. Accessed January 28, 2016.
57. Hardy MS. Teaching firearm safety to children: failure of a program. J Dev Behav Pediatr 2002;23(2):71–6.
58. Connor SM, Wesolowski KL. "They're too smart for that": predicting what children would do in the presence of guns. Pediatrics 2003;111(2):E109–14.
59. Jackman GA, Farah MM, Kellermann AL, et al. Seeing is believing: what do boys do when they find a real gun? Pediatrics 2001;107(6):1247–50.
60. Baxley F, Miller M. Parental misperceptions about children and firearms. Arch Pediatr Adolesc Med 2006;160(5):542–7.
61. Farah MM, Simon HK, Kellermann AL. Firearms in the home: parental perceptions. Pediatrics 1999;104(5 Pt 1):1059–63.
62. Webster DW, Wilson ME, Duggan AK, et al. Parents' beliefs about preventing gun injuries to children. Pediatrics 1992;89(5 Pt 1):908–14.
63. Miller M, Hemenway D. Unsupervised firearm handling by California adolescents. Inj Prev 2004;10(3):163–8.
64. United States of America, Plaintiff-Appellee v. Gilbert Martinez-Jimenez, Defendant-Appellant. 1989. Available at: http://openjurist.org/864/f2d/664/united-states-v-martinez-jimenez. Accessed April 3, 2016.
65. Wood RH. Toy guns don't kill people - people kill people who play with toy guns: federal attempts to regulate imitation firearms in the face of toy industry opposition. New York City L Rev 2009;12(2):263–82. Available at: http://heinonline.org/HOL/Page?handle=hein.journals/nyclr12&div=16&g_sent=1&collection=journals. Accessed April 16, 2016.
66. Carlson K, Fin P. Test of the visibility of toy and replica handgun markings. Cambridge, MA: Abt Associates, Inc; 1989. Available at: https://www.ncjrs.gov/pdffiles1/digitization/146870NCJRS.pdf. Accessed March 27, 2016.
67. Carter DL, Sapp AD, Stephens DW. Toy guns: involvement in crime and encounters with the police. Washington, DC: Police Executive Research Forum; 1990. Available at: http:www/bjs.gov/content/pub/pdf/tg-icep.pdf. Accessed March 27, 2016.
68. STAFF CC. Toy gun forces airport lockdown. CBSNEWS.com. 2000. Available at: http://www.cbsnews.com/news/toy-gun-forces-airport-lockdown/. Accessed November 21, 2000.
69. The Council Of The City Of New York. Toy guns: a deadly game. 2003. Available at: http://www.nyc.gov/html/records/pdf/govpub/838toyguns.pdf. Accessed March 27, 2016.
70. Dowd MD, Sege RD. Firearm-related injuries affecting the pediatric population. Pediatrics 2012;130(5):e1416–23.
71. Okoro CA, Nelson DE, Mercy JA, et al. Prevalence of household firearms and firearm-storage practices in the 50 states and the District of Columbia: findings from the Behavioral Risk Factor Surveillance System, 2002. Pediatrics 2005;116(3):e370–6.
72. Hepburn L, Azrael D, Miller M, et al. The effect of child access prevention laws on unintentional child firearm fatalities, 1979-2000. J Trauma 2006;61(2):423–8.
73. Webster DW, Starnes M. Reexamining the association between child access prevention gun laws and unintentional shooting deaths of children. Pediatrics 2000;106(6):1466–9.

74. Cummings P, Grossman DC, Rivara FP, et al. State gun safe storage laws and child mortality due to firearms. JAMA 1997;278(13):1084–6.
75. Prickett KC, Martin-Storey A, Crosnoe R. State firearm laws, firearm ownership, and safety practices among families of preschool-aged children. Am J Public Health 2014;104(6):1080–6.
76. Barkin SL, Finch SA, Ip EH, et al. Is office-based counseling about media use, timeouts, and firearm storage effective? Results from a cluster-randomized, controlled trial. Pediatrics 2008;122(1):e15–25.
77. Grossman DC, Cummings P, Koepsell TD, et al. Firearm safety counseling in primary care pediatrics: a randomized, controlled trial. Pediatrics 2000;106(1):22–6.

Increased Screen Time
Implications for Early Childhood Development and Behavior

Jenny S. Radesky, MD[a],*, Dimitri A. Christakis, MD, MPH[b]

KEYWORDS

- Television • Digital media • Mobile device • Screen time • Child behavior
- Child development • Child play

KEY POINTS

- Mobile and interactive media have revolutionized digital play for young children, through changes in access to platforms, new content, and differences in the ways parents mediate this play.
- Well-designed TV programs and interactive media can be educational starting in pre-school; but children younger than 2 years require adult interaction to learn from screen media.
- Interactive media have the potential to be highly engaging for children, but digital features can also distract from the learning objectives.
- Several health and developmental risks of excessive or inappropriate (eg, violent, adult oriented) media exposure continue to exist, primarily in areas of sleep, obesity, child development, executive functioning, and aggression.
- Pediatric providers can be a resource for parents in terms of translating these research findings and applying them to family's decision-making, offering suggestions for digital tools or resources, teaching parents how to mediate their child's screen time, and supporting positive parenting and play.

INTRODUCTION

Emerging technologies, including mobile and interactive screen media, are now embedded in the daily lives of young children.[1,2] Since 1970, the age at which children begin to regularly interact with media has shifted from 4 years to 4 months, meaning that children today are "digital natives," born into an ever-changing digital ecosystem that is enhanced by mobile media. Although there have been decades of research on the effects of TV on children's health and development, there is considerably less research on more recent platforms, including interactive and mobile media.

[a] University of Michigan Medical School, University of Michigan, 300 North Ingalls Street, Suite 1107, Ann Arbor, MI 48108, USA; [b] CW8-6 Child Health, Behavior and Development, 2001 Eighth Avenue, Seattle, WA 98121, USA
* Corresponding author.
E-mail address: jradesky@umich.edu

Pediatr Clin N Am 63 (2016) 827–839
http://dx.doi.org/10.1016/j.pcl.2016.06.006
0031-3955/16/$ – see front matter © 2016 Elsevier Inc. All rights reserved.

In this article, the authors review the evidence of how young children learn through digital media in different domains of child development and learning as well as evidence for developmental risks. This article focuses on early childhood and school-aged children (approximately 0–8 years of age), when lifelong media habits are established,[3] before children are usually using social media, and when parents play the largest role in determining children's media use habits. This time is also a period of enormous brain plasticity, when experiences exert profound influences on social, cognitive, and emotional development[4,5] and when health-related behaviors, such as eating, physical activity, and sleep, are established.

HOW DIGITAL MEDIA USE IS CHANGING
Increasing Use, Younger Ages

Digital media is increasingly used by children during these early years of brain development. This increased use reflects both the increasing use of screen media by families and society[6] and the growing marketing of cable TV channels, digital devices, and applications (apps) to young children,[7] even to those from disadvantaged households.[8]

For example, since the Kaiser Family Foundation first started surveying parents of 0 to 8 year olds about family technology use, usage by young children has increased year by year. In 2011, 52% of children aged 0 to 8 years had access to a mobile device and 38% had ever used one.[9] This percentage increased to 75% of 0- to 8-year-old children having access to mobile devices in 2013.[6] At that point, most mobile device use was reportedly to play games, use apps, or watch videos, averaging only 15 minutes per day. Children younger than 2 years were primarily still watching TV and DVDs.[6]

Since then, a nationwide survey showed that 0 to 8 year olds are using an average of 3 hours of screen media per day (**Table 1**), primarily watching TV or videos.[2] A smaller study conducted in a low-income urban pediatric clinic in 2015 showed that almost all (97%) 0 to 4 year olds had used a mobile device, and three-quarters owned their own device.[8] What is even more striking about these results is evidence that media multitasking starts at less than 4 years of age, that the youngest children queried had almost universal exposure to mobile devices in infancy (92% of 1 year olds), and that most young children were primarily using mobile devices for entertainment, not educational, purposes.

Table 1
Average time spent using screen media by children at home per day, by age

	Among All	Younger than 2 y	2–5 y	6–8 y
TV or DVDs	1:46	0:59	2:01	1:52
Computer	0:25	0:09	0:20	0:42
Video game player (console)	0:18	-	0:14	0:31
Tablet computer	0:14	0:02	0:16	0:17
Handheld video game player	0:11	0:01	0:10	0:18
Smartphone	0:10	0:03	0:13	0:11
Total	3:04	1:15	3:13	3:52

From Wartella E, Rideout V, Lauricella A, et al. Parenting in the age of digital technology: a national survey. Report of the Center on Media and Human Development, School of Communication, Northwestern University. 2014.

Changing Content

Although apps and games created for children have been the fastest growing section of app stores,[10] their usage has been hard to accurately measure in research studies. Most parents report that their young children stream videos or play apps and games on mobile devices.[7,9] For example, in Kabali and colleagues[8] (2015) most children were reported to primarily watch YouTube or Netflix, whereas smaller proportions watched educational TV programs, played educational apps, or played games.

Parent Mediation Is More Challenging

With these changes in content, it is even more important that parents monitor what their children are consuming and help them learn from it, which has long been recommended for TV and videos.[11] However, many parents report that mobile devices, which are handheld and usually used individually, are more difficult to monitor in terms of what the child is playing or downloading as well as where and when they are using media.[12] Instant accessibility now means that children can demand preferred programs at any time or place. For example, Hiniker and colleagues[13] surveyed parents of children and teens and found that *context-based rules* (ie, where children are allowed to use digital media, such as the dinner table) were the hardest to enforce compared with rules about time limits and content (**Fig. 1**).

The Changing Digital Divide

Although the digital divide between higher- and lower-income families has been narrowed in terms of mobile technology ownership,[1] disparities still exist in many domains. For example, in a national survey of families, Wartella[2] found that low-income families were more likely to be the media-centric families (**Table 2**) whose households are saturated with background media throughout the day, which is known to disrupt child play and interactions with parents.[14,15] A recent survey by the Joan Ganz Cooney Center at Sesame Workshop found that digital resources were usually not well guided to ensure educational progress in low-income communities.[16] Similarly, the 2013 Zero to Eight survey found disparities in use of educational mobile media by income; 54%

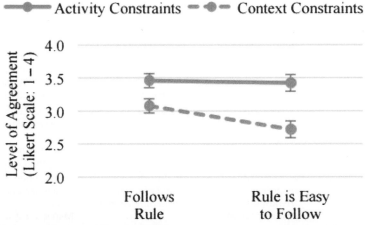

Fig. 1. Parents' reported ability to enforce screen time rules at home. (*From* Hiniker A, Schoenebeck S, Kientz J. Not at the dinner table: parents' and children's perspectives on family technology rules. CSCW '16 Proceedings of the 19th ACM Conference on Computer-Supported Cooperative Work & Social Computing, pages 1376-1389; with permission.)

Table 2
Use of individual screen media among media-centric, media-moderate, and media-light parents of 0 to 8 year olds

	Media-Light Parents	Media-Moderate Parents	Media-Centric Parents
TV or DVDs	0:54	2:12	4:19
Computer	0:34	1:26	3:35
Video games	0:03	0:12	0:36
iPad, iPod touch, or similar device	0:07	0:19	0:36
Smartphone	0:10	0:34	1:57
Total screen media use	1:48	4:42	11:03

From Wartella E, Rideout V, Lauricella A, et al. Parenting in the age of digital technology: a national survey. Report of the Center on Media and Human Development, School of Communication, Northwestern University. 2014.

of higher income children often or sometimes used educational content on mobile devices, whereas only 28% of lower income children did.[6]

ARE NEWER DIGITAL MEDIA EDUCATIONAL? AFFORDANCES AND LIMITATIONS
Cognitive Development

The ability of young children to learn from screen media is largely age dependent (**Table 3**). For children younger than 2 years, when children are still in Piaget's sensorimotor stage of development, their understanding of content on 2-dimensional screens is limited. For example, infants can imitate and recall actions performed by

Table 3
Examples of child development and learning domains that may or may not be supported effectively by digital products

	High Yield	Possible Yield	Unlikely Yield/Possible Detriment
Cognitive	Skill-and-drill concepts (math, rote facts) Videos/visual illustrations of new concepts	Executive function training (unclear if generalizes) Problem-solving (within close-ended problem)	Creative problem-solving Concern for multitasking and attention span Tolerance of boredom/brain downtime
Language/literacy	Skill-and-drill training (letters, phonemic awareness, sight words, vocabulary)	Comprehension (if digital interface is not distracting)	Early word learning (<2 y) Conversational/pragmatic language
Social-emotional	Prosocial content regarding friendships, feelings, polite behavior	Social stories, self-regulation apps to prompt relaxation	Reading nonverbal cues/perspective taking Managing strong emotions in the moment Displacement of family routines

a person on a screen[17] or imitate sign language from videos[18] but cannot learn new knowledge (eg, novel words, solve puzzles) at less than 30 months of age without a real-life adult helping them learn.[19] At this age, it is thought that attentional controls and symbolic thinking are too immature for children to be able to transfer knowledge from screen to 3-dimensional life.[20]

Although it is possible that the interactivity of touch screens may make them more educational for infants and toddlers, research has only shown that children as young as 24 months can learn from videochat[21] or carefully designed touch screens.[22] No research has been conducted on children younger than 2 years as of yet. However, it is worth noting that the interactivity of touch screens is limited compared with teaching from an adult. Adults are able to read and respond contingently to the knowledge, behavior, and affective state of children to be able to teach them on their learning edge—what Vygotsky (1978)[23] termed the *zone of proximal development*—where the greatest amount of learning can occur. Even the most tailored educational apps and games do not have this complex capacity.

Higher-Order Thinking: the Executive Functions

Executive functions, which start to develop at about 4 years of age but are rooted in experiences as early as infancy, predict early school success[24] and college graduation rates independent of intelligence.[25] Executive functions, such as task persistence, impulse control, emotion regulation, and creative, flexible thinking, are influenced through positive parenting[26] as well as child-led play[27]; but a growing body of literature is examining whether brain training computer games can improve these mental capacities. In children aged 6 years and older, there is early evidence that intensive computerized working memory training may be effective for children with attention-deficit/hyperactivity disorder (ADHD)[28] or prematurity.[29] However, results are conflicting.[30] Experts in the field have warned that children may not generalize such digital skills to their everyday environments[31] or that the closed-loop of app-based learning teaches less critical thinking.[32]

Language and Literacy

A large body of research has examined whether high-quality educational programming can teach children language and early literacy skills. As noted earlier, children younger than 2.5 years cannot learn novel words from videos without parents coviewing and using the same words in everyday interactions.[33,34] However, by preschool age, well-designed traditional[35,36] and interactive educational digital media can teach children language and literacy skills.[37] Similarly, studies show that children learn content knowledge and vocabulary equally from digital books and print books, as long as formal features of the digital books support the learning objectives, rather than distract from them.[38]

However, it is important to understand whether the use of digital books engages children in more solo reading, at the expense of shared parent-child reading experiences. Some studies show that, when reading digital books with young children, parents use fewer dialogic reading strategies, such as labeling objects, asking open-ended questions, and commenting on the story beyond the actual pictures, but instead comment on the digital device itself (eg, tap that…push this).[33] Because active parent involvement in digital play or e-book reading improves children's learning,[39,40] it is important that shared parent-child experiences not be displaced.

Social-Emotional Development

Play is central to child social-emotional development because it provides a special opportunity for affective exchanges and enriched experiences between parents and children.[41] It allows parents a window into their child's thoughts and conflicts, lets them follow the child's lead, and, thus, builds social reciprocity. However, background TV has been shown to distract from parent-child interaction[16,42] and child play.[15] This distraction has been proposed as one of the mechanisms by which screen exposure negatively influences child social-emotional development (see section on child development).

However, certain forms of digital play or creation may be effective at bringing a parent into a child's world, for example, a child taking photos or videos and then showing them to a parent, or audio recording/illustrating stories together. Regarding social skills, evidence shows that quality TV programs, such as *Sesame Street* and *Mister Rogers' Neighborhood*, improve children's understanding of concepts, including friendship, feelings, and how to treat other people.[16,17] Although some interactive apps have been developed to promote social-emotional skills, none have been formally tested.

Summing Up: The Importance of Adult Interaction and Good Digital Design

For infants and toddlers younger than 24 to 30 months, the primary way children learn from passive or interactive media is through caregivers coviewing, teaching them about the content, and repeating this teaching through daily interactions. Thus, any digital media product that does not try to involve the caregiver is unlikely to be educational at these younger ages.

In preschoolers, well-designed educational apps based on established curricula can be educational[32]; but most of the commercially available apps marketed as educational have no evidence to back up this claim. In fact, recent reviews of the most popular or highest-rated educational apps in iTunes showed that most have no input from developmental scientists, are not based on curricula, and target only simple skills (eg, colors, ABCs).[8,43] Thus, academic and industry leaders have recently issued recommendations for app design that include (1) fewer distracting features, so that children can truly engage with learning content; (2) design for a dual audience (ie, both parent and child) to facilitate family participation in media use[8]; and (3) features that allow the child to transfer their knowledge to the physical and social world around them.[44]

DEVELOPMENTAL AND BEHAVIORAL RISKS

Potential negative effects of screen media on child health have been the subject of study for the past 30 years, focusing on the areas of child development, aggressive behavior, obesity, and sleep. Although little has been studied regarding links between mobile or interactive media and these outcomes, it is reasonable to extrapolate findings from TV or videos to these newer media platforms.

Child Development

Population-based reports have shown associations of excessive TV viewing in early childhood with cognitive,[45–47] language,[48,49] and social/emotional delays.[50–53] This is thought to be due to effects of inappropriate, adult-oriented content,[34] displacement of parent-child interaction,[42] and overall poorer family functioning.[40]

Newer evidence suggests that some young children develop excessive media habits as a parenting response to their difficult behaviors: excessive media use is more likely in infants and toddlers with difficult temperament[54,55] or self-regulation problems.[56] In addition, low-income toddlers with social-emotional delays are more likely to be given a mobile device to calm them down or keep them quiet.[57]

Longer-term relationships between child temperament and media use need to be understood.

Executive Functioning and Attention

Building on earlier reports linking excessive early childhood media use to ADHD risk,[58] recent studies have shown associations between early childhood media use and poorer executive functioning. These studies show that earlier age of media use onset, greater cumulative hours of media use, and non–Public Broadcasting Service content are all significant independent predictors of poor executive functioning.[59,60] This relationship has been attributed to both the stimulating and fast-paced content of some children's programming[61] and to the displacement of other enriching activities or brain downtime.

Media multitasking, which itself is associated with executive functioning deficits in young adults,[62] has now been documented in children as young as 4 years of age.[8] The visual and sound effects of apps and TV shows may be particularly attention grabbing in younger children,[63] but it is unknown whether rapid shifts in attention to and from digital stimuli have long-term effects on child executive functions.

Aggressive Behavior and Problematic Video Gaming

Robust associations between violent media content and child aggressive behavior have been documented,[64] thought to be due to children imitating on-screen behavior and arousal responses to frightening content. Decreasing violent media viewing is also a promising avenue for intervention; Christakis and colleagues[36] showed that, by replacing violent media with educational and prosocial programming, preschoolers' externalizing and social behaviors could be improved significantly, even without changes in overall screen time. These effects were particularly strong in low-income boys.

Now that violent content is also contained in numerous violent and first-person aggression video games, young children are often exposed in families with older siblings. Problematic gaming is well described in older children[65,66]; however, it is unknown how early problematic gaming habits develop or what children are most at risk of developing them.

Sleep

It is well documented that having a TV in a child's bedroom is associated with poorer sleep quality and quantity; but the same is true for all screen media, primarily because of later bedtimes after evening media use.[67] Some have attributed this to suppression of endogenous melatonin from light emitted by screens[68] as well as due to overstimulation and arousing content.[69] Later onset of sleep after evening media exposure has been documented in infants[70] as well as older children. This association has been found to be stronger in racial/ethnic minority children.[71]

Background/Parent Media Use

Parent media use is strongly correlated with child media habits[72] and, therefore, has received attention as a potential point of intervention not only for how parents role model media use for children but also its displacement of parent-child engagement. As noted earlier, background TV distracts from parent-child interactions[16] and play[15]; but parent mobile device use may do the same.[73] Preliminary studies have also suggested more parent-child conflict when parents' attention is absorbed in mobile devices[74] and less effective parent-child teaching when parents are interrupted by their phones.[75]

HEALTH RISKS
Obesity

Heavy media use during the preschool and early school-aged years is associated with increases in body mass index (BMI),[76] and this association persists even after adjusting for children's psychosocial risk factors or behavioral problems.[77] Of even greater public health relevance is the finding that media use habits may explain some of the disparities in obesity risk among minority race/ethnicity children.[78] One study in 2 year olds found that even a 1-hour-per-week increase in total media consumption predicted increases in BMI, suggesting that limits more conservative than 2 hours per day might be needed for obesity prevention.[79] None of these studies specifically examined mobile media, which can be brought to meals more easily and contain advertising that is more difficult to regulate.[80]

DISCUSSION: CLINICAL IMPLICATIONS

Parents frequently voice uncertainty regarding how to adopt new technologies in their families, and it can be difficult for pediatric providers' knowledge to keep pace with rapid developments in platforms and content. However, it is worth understanding the tensions parents face about their children's use of new technologies (**Box 1**), because clinic-based counseling is one of the few effective interventional strategies for changing screen time habits.[81]

Specifically, pediatricians have a vital role to play in helping parents identify good versus less-optimal content and digital tools that will help them monitor, coview, limit, and reinforce what is learned from screen time (**Box 2**). Having rules about where children and parents can use media (eg, bedroom, dinner table) is just as important as rules about content and time limits. Most importantly, pediatricians can help parents understand they are important role models for digital media habits and have the power to teach their children to connect and create, rather than consume, and then to be able to transition off of digital play. Advice on achieving this goal may include suggesting alternative activities that meet the same family goals. Given the potential benefits of digital technology as a tool to enhance early childhood development, creativity, and social connection, it is important that parents proactively think about using media

---

Box 1
Suggested points of discussion between pediatric providers and parents of young children about digital media use

- What rules do they have for family media use (for both parents and children)?
- What are the child's favorite apps and tablet activities? Is it mostly passive or interactive?
- Do parents and children use technology in creative ways?
- Do the parents worry about how much their child uses or demands technology?
- Do the parents feel empowered to set limits on media use?
- Where do they get information about apps, programs, and movies?
- Do the parents need ideas for alternate activities?

> **Box 2**
> **Recommendations about healthy media use practices for families with young children**
>
> - Do not allow screen media during family meals, bedtime (turn off 1 hour before bed), or playtime (unless playing on the device together).
> - Watch and play with digital media together.
> - Help the child apply any knowledge gained from apps or TV programs to the rest of their life.
> - Check out which apps the child is downloading and uninstall those that are violent or inappropriate.
> - Suggest resources, such as www.commonsensemedia.org, Sesame Workshop, or PBS Kids, which all provide good guidance for parents.
> - Ensure adequate time in physical activity, hands-on play, social play, and sleep.
> - Create an American Academy of Pediatrics' Family Media Use Plan that fits with your family's goals and needs.

for these purposes while also preserving time for unplugged learning, physical, social, and emotional experiences.

REFERENCES

1. Pew Internet Research Center. Technology adoption by lower income populations. 2015. Available at: http://www.pewinternet.org/2013/10/08/technology-adoption-by-lower-income-populations/. Accessed April 1, 2016.
2. Wartella E, Rideout V, Lauricella AR, et al. Parenting in the age of digital technology. Chicago: Northwestern University Press; 2014.
3. Zimmerman FJ, Christakis DA, Meltzoff AN. Television and DVD/video viewing in children younger than 2 years. Arch Pediatr Adolesc Med 2007;161(5):473–9.
4. Jimenez ME, Wade R Jr, Lin Y, et al. Adverse experiences in early childhood and kindergarten outcomes. Pediatrics 2016;137:1–9.
5. Wade R Jr, Cronholm PF, Fein JA, et al. Household and community-level adverse childhood experiences and adult health outcomes in a diverse urban population. Child Abuse Negl 2016;52:135–45.
6. Rideout V. Zero to eight: children's media use in America 2013: a Common Sense Media research study. Common Sense Media. Available at: www.commonsensemedia.org. Accessed April 1, 2016.
7. Vaala S, Ly A, Levine M. Getting a read on the app stores: a market scan and analysis of children's literacy apps. New York: The Joan Ganz Cooney Center at Sesame Workshop; 2015. Available at: http://www.joanganzcooneycenter.org/wp-content/uploads/2015/12/jgcc_gettingaread.pdf.
8. Kabali H, Irigoyen M, Nunez-Davis R, et al. Exposure to and use of mobile devices by young children. Pediatrics 2015;136(6):1044–50.
9. Rideout V. Zero to eight: children's media use in America 2011. Common Sense Media. Available at: www.commonsensemedia.org. Accessed April 1, 2016.
10. Schuler C. iLearnII: an analysis of the education category on Apple's app store. New York: The Joan Ganz Cooney Center at Sesame Workshop; 2012. Available at: http://www.joanganzcooneycenter.org/publication/ilearn-ii-an-analysis-of-the-education-category-on-apples-app-store/.
11. Strasburger VC, Hogan MJ, Mulligan DA, et al. Children, adolescents, and the media. Pediatrics 2013;132(5):958–61.

12. Radesky JS, Eisenberg S, Kistin CJ, et al. Overstimulated consumers or next-generation learners? Parent tensions about child mobile technology use. Annals of Family Medicine, in press.

13. Hiniker A, Schoenebeck SY, Kientz JA. Not at the dinner table: parents' and children's perspectives on family technology rules. CSCW '16, ACM. San Francisco, February 27, 2016. http://dx.doi.org/10.1145/2818048.2819940.

14. Schmidt ME, Pempek TA, Kirkorian HL, et al. The effects of background television on the toy play behavior of very young children. Child Dev 2008;79(4):1137–51.

15. Kirkorian HL, Pempek TA, Murphy LA, et al. The impact of background television on parent-child interaction. Child Dev 2009;80(5):1350–9.

16. Rideout V, Katz V. Opportunity for all? Technology and learning in lower-income families. New York: The Joan Ganz Cooney Center at Sesame Workshop; 2016. Available at: http://www.joanganzcooneycenter.org/publication/opportunity-for-all-technology-and-learning-in-lower-income-families/.

17. Barr R, Muentener P, Garcia A. Age-related changes in deferred imitation from television by 6- to 18-month-olds. Dev Sci 2007;10(6):910–21.

18. Dayanim S, Namy LL. Infants learn baby signs from video. Child Dev 2015;86(3): 800–11.

19. Dickerson K, Gerhardstein P, Zack E, et al. Age-related changed in learning across early childhood: a new imitation task. Dev Psychobiol 2013;55(7):719–32.

20. Courage ML, Howe ML. To watch or not to watch: infants and toddlers in a brave new electronic world. Dev Rev 2010;30:101–15.

21. Roseberry S, Hirsh-Pasek K, Golinkoff RM. Skype me! Socially contingent interactions help toddlers learn language. Child Dev 2014;85(3):956–70.

22. Kirkorian H, Choi K, Pempek T. Toddlers' word learning from contingent and non-contingent video on touchscreens. Child Dev 2016;87:405–13.

23. Vygotsky L. Mind and Society. Cambridge, MA: Harvard University Press; 1978.

24. Blair C, Razza RP. Relating effortful control, executive function, and false belief understanding to emerging math and literacy ability in kindergarten. Child Dev 2007;78(2):647–63.

25. McClelland MM, Acock AC, Piccinin A, et al. Relations between preschool attention span-persistence and age 25 educational outcomes. Early Child Res Q 2013; 28(2):314–24.

26. Blair C, Granger DA, Willoughby M, et al, FLP Investigators. Salivary cortisol mediates effects of poverty and parenting on executive functions in early childhood. Child Dev 2011;82(6):1970–84.

27. Shaheen S. How child's play impacts executive function-related behaviors. Appl Neuropsychol Child 2014;3(3):182–7.

28. Bigorra A, Garolera M, Guijarro S, et al. Long-term far-transfer effects of working memory training in children with ADHD: a randomized controlled trial. Eur Child Adolesc Psychiatry 2015;15:1–5.

29. Grunewaldt KH, Skranes J, Brubakk AM, et al. Computerized working memory training has positive long-term effect in very low birthweight preschool children. Dev Med Child Neurol 2016;58:195–201.

30. Rode C, Robson R, Purviance A, et al. Is working memory training effective? A study in a school setting. PLoS One 2014;9(8):e104796.

31. Diamond A, Lee K. Interventions shown to aid executive function development in children 4 to 12 years old. Science 2009;333:959–63.

32. Greenfield P. Technology and informal education: what is taught, what is learned. Science 2009;323:69–71.

33. Deloache JS, Chiong C, Sherman K, et al. Do babies learn from baby media? Psychol Sci 2010;21(11):1570–4.
34. Richert RA, Robb MB, Fender JG, et al. Word learning from baby videos. Arch Pediatr Adolesc Med 2010;164(5):432–7.
35. Anderson DR, Huston AC, Schmitt KL, et al. Early childhood television viewing and adolescent behavior: the recontact study. Monogr Soc Res Child Dev 2001;66(1):1–147.
36. Christakis DA, Garrison MM, Herrenkohl T, et al. Modifying media content for preschool children: a randomized controlled trial. Pediatrics 2013;131(3):431–8.
37. Chiong C, Shuler C. Learning: is there an app for that? Investigations of young children's usage and learning with mobile devices and apps. New York: The Joan Ganz Cooney Center at Sesame Workshop; 2010. Available at: http://www-tc.pbskids.org/read/files/cooney_learning_apps.pdf.
38. Bus AG, Takacs ZK, Kegel CA. Affordances and limitations of electronic storybooks for young children's emergent literacy. Dev Rev 2015;35:79–97.
39. Lauricella AR, Barr R, Calvert S. Parent-child interactions during traditional and computer storybook reading predict children's story comprehension. Int J Child Comput Interact 2014. http://dx.doi.org/10.1016/j.ijcci.2014.07.001.
40. Strouse GA, O'Doherty K, Troseth GL. Effective coviewing: preschoolers' learning from video after a dialogic questioning intervention. Dev Psychol 2013;49(12):2368–82.
41. Ginsberg K, American Academy of Pediatrics Committee on Communications, American Academy of Pediatrics Committee on Psychosocial Aspects of Child and Family Health. The importance of play in promoting healthy child development and maintaining strong parent-child bonds. Pediatrics 2007;119(1):182–91.
42. Christakis DA, Gillkerson J, Richards JA, et al. Audible television and decreased adult words, infant vocalizations, and conversational turns: a population-based study. Arch Pediatr Adolesc Med 2009;163(6):554–8.
43. Guernsey L, Levine MH. Tap click read: growing readers in a world of screens. San Francisco (CA): Jossey-Bass; 2015.
44. Hirsh-Pasek K, Zosh JM, Golinkoff RM, et al. Putting education in "educational" apps: lessons from the science of learning. Psychol Sci Public Interest 2015;16(1):3–34.
45. Tomopoulos S, Dreyer BP, Berkule S, et al. Infant media exposure and toddler development. Arch Pediatr Adolesc Med 2010;164(12):1105–11.
46. Schmidt ME, Rich M, Rifas-Shiman SL, et al. Television viewing in infancy and child cognition at 3 years of age in a US cohort. Pediatrics 2009;123(3):e370–5.
47. Lin LY, Cherng RJ, Chen YJ, et al. Effects of television exposure on developmental skills among young children. Infant Behav Dev 2015;38:20–6.
48. Zimmerman FJ, Christakis DA, Meltzoff AN. Associations between media viewing and language development in children under age 2 years. J Pediatr 2007;151:364–8.
49. Duch H, Fisher EM, Ensari I, et al. Association of screen time use and language development in Hispanic toddlers: a cross-sectional and longitudinal study. Clin Pediatr 2013;52(9):857–65.
50. Tomopoulos S, Dreyer BP, Valdez P, et al. Media content and externalizing behaviors in Latino toddlers. Ambul Pediatr 2007;7(3):232–8.
51. Hinkley T, Verbestel V, Ahrens W, et al. Early childhood electronic media use as a predictor of poorer well-being: a prospective cohort study. JAMA Pediatr 2014;168(5):485–92.

52. Pagani LS, Fitzpatrick C, Barnett TA, et al. Prospective associations between early childhood television exposure and academic, psychosocial, and physical well-being by middle childhood. Arch Pediatr Adolesc Med 2010;164(5):425–31.

53. Conners-Burrow NA, McKelvey LM, Fussell JJ. Social outcomes associated with media viewing habits of low-income preschool children. Early Educ Dev 2011;22: 256–73.

54. Thompson AL, Adair LS, Bentley ME. Maternal characteristics and perception of temperament associated with infant TV exposure. Pediatrics 2013;131(2):e390–7.

55. Sugawara M, Matsumoto S, Murohashi H, et al. Trajectories of early television contact in Japan: relationship with preschoolers' externalizing problems. J Child Media 2015;9(4):453–71.

56. Radesky JS, Silverstein M, Zuckerman B, et al. Infant self-regulation and early childhood media exposure. Pediatrics 2014;133(5):e1172–8.

57. Radesky JS, Peacock-Chambers E, Zuckerman B, et al. Use of Mobile Technology to Calm Upset Children: Associations With Social-Emotional Development. JAMA pediatrics 2016;170(4):397–9.

58. Christakis DA, Zimmerman FJ, DiGiuseppe DL, et al. Early television exposure and subsequent attentional problems in children. Pediatrics 2004;113(4):708–13.

59. Nathanson AI, Alade F, Sharp ML, et al. The relation between television exposure and executive function among preschoolers. Dev Psychol 2014;50(5):1497–506.

60. Barr R, Lauricella A, Zack E, et al. Infant and early childhood exposure to adult directed and child-directed television programming: relations with cognitive skills at age four. Merrill Palmer Q 2010;56(1):21–48.

61. Lillard AS, Peterson J. The immediate impact of different types of television on young children's executive function. Pediatrics 2011;128(4):644–9.

62. Minear M, Brasher F, McCurdy M, et al. Working memory, fluid intelligence, and impulsiveness in heavy media multitaskers. Psychon Bull Rev 2013;20(6): 1274–81.

63. Rothbart MK, Posner MI. The developing brain in a multitasking world. Dev Rev 2015;1(35):42–63.

64. Christakis DA. AAP Council on Communications and Media. Virtual violence policy statement. Pediatrics, in press.

65. Christakis DA, Moreno MM, Jelenchick L, et al. Problematic Internet usage in US college students: a pilot study. BMC Med 2011;9:77.

66. Grusser SM, Thalemann R, Griffiths MD. Excessive computer game playing: evidence for addiction and aggression? Cyberpsychol Behav 2007;10(2):290–2.

67. McDonald L, Wardle J, Llewellyn CH, et al. Predictors of shorter sleep in early childhood. Sleep Med 2014;15(5):536–40.

68. Salti R, Tarquini R, Stagi S, et al. Age-dependent association of exposure to television screen with children's urinary melatonin excretion? Neuro Endocrinol Lett 2006;27(1–2):73–80.

69. Garrison MM, Christakis DA. The impact of a healthy media use intervention on sleep in preschool children. Pediatrics 2012;130(3):492–9.

70. Vijakkhana N, Wilaisakditipakorn T, Ruedeekhajorn K, et al. Evening media exposure reduces nighttime sleep. Acta Paediatr 2015;104(3):306–12.

71. Cespedes EM, Gillman MW, Kleinman K, et al. Television viewing, bedroom television, and sleep duration from infancy to mid-childhood. Pediatrics 2014;133(5): e1163–71.

72. Jago R, Stamatakis E, Gama A, et al. Parent and child screen-viewing time and home media environment. Am J Prev Med 2012;43(2):150–8.

73. Radesky JS, Miller AL, Rosenblum KL, et al. Maternal mobile device use during a parent-child interaction task. Acad Pediatr 2015;15(2):238–44.
74. Radesky JS, Kistin CJ, Zuckerman B, et al. Patterns of mobile device use by caregivers and young children during meals in fast food restaurants. Pediatrics 2014; 133(4):e843–9.
75. Reed J, Hirsh-Pasek K, Golinkoff RM. Learning on hold: cell phones sidetrack parent-child interactions, in press.
76. Cox R, Skouteris H, Rutherford L, et al. Television viewing, television content, food intake, physical activity and body mass index: a cross-sectional study of preschool children aged 2-6 years. Health Promot J Austr 2012;23(1):58–62.
77. Suglia SF, Duarte CS, Chambers EC, et al. Social and behavioral risk factors for obesity in early childhood. J Dev Behav Pediatr 2013;34(8):549–56.
78. Taveras EM, Gillman MW, Kleinman KP, et al. Reducing racial/ethnic disparities in childhood obesity: the role of early life risk factors. JAMA Pediatr 2013;167(8): 731–8.
79. Wen LM, Baur LA, Rissel C, et al. Correlates of body mass index and overweight and obesity of children aged 2 years: findings from the healthy beginnings trial. Obesity 2014;22(7):1723–30.
80. Zimmerman FJ, Bell JF. Associations of television content type and obesity in children. Am J Public Health 2010;100(2):334–400.
81. Schmidt ME, Haines J, O'Brien A, et al. Systematic review of effective strategies for reducing screen time among young children. Obesity 2012;20(7):1338–54.

Social Media

Challenges and Concerns for Families

Gwenn Schurgin O'Keeffe, MD

KEYWORDS

- Social media • Cyber-bullying • Sexting • Family media plan • Texting
- Applications • Games

KEY POINTS

- Social media is everywhere and used by adults and children.
- Social media can have a positive impact on child development in terms of fostering communication, socialization, and learning.
- Social medial can have a negative impact on child development with such issues as bullying, sexting, and inappropriate content contributing to additional issues.
- Social media can have positive and negative issues on family health and needs to be used within a family with attention and care with a focus on the ages of the children at home.

INTRODUCTION

"What's the harm?" That's the age-old rhetorical question parents ask when trying to convince themselves that the new shiny toy or gizmo on the block is safe for their children. In the age of electronics, this question has been asked about every new device: video cassette recorders, televisions, radios, Walkmen, MP3 players, cell phones used as phones, smart phones, tablets, gaming systems, apps, and now social media. As with issues in the nondigital world, safety with social media is a balance between common sense and understanding the rules of what one is using. Social media is a tool. Like all tools, whether there is harm or not depends on how it is used. Used correctly, there should not be a need for concern. Used incorrectly, problems could arise.

Technology is faceless so it is tempting to forget that issues can occur from its use. Technology seems like a mere tool, an extension of the ability to connect and communicate. With a device in hand, we forget that there are people at the other end. With interactions with people, however, complications can arise from miscommunications to true harm, such as privacy breaches and bullying.

With face-to-face connections, we are not so brazen. We take more care in how we interact. We are careful in our choice of words and our mannerisms. We teach our

Pediatrics Now, PO Box 5336, Wayland, MA 01778, USA
E-mail address: DrGwenn@pediatricsnow.com

Pediatr Clin N Am 63 (2016) 841–849
http://dx.doi.org/10.1016/j.pcl.2016.06.009
0031-3955/16/$ – see front matter © 2016 Elsevier Inc. All rights reserved.

children the social norms and behaviors expected for negotiating the world. We do not allow our children into certain situations until they are old enough. Some of these situations we determine, but others are determined by society, such as the drinking age and driving age.

So, why do we allow our children to use social media sites, such as Facebook, Instagram, Kik, Twitter, and others, before their privacy policies allow? Why do we let them lie about their ages to use these sites? What is it about technology that lets us bend these rules in a way we would never do in the unplugged world?

Gaining insight into the answers to these questions and what is positive and negative about social media and the digital world allows us to talk to families about this world, allay their concerns, and keep children of all age safe when using social media. We live in a social media–focused world, a world that will only become more digitally connected. Our job is to help parents stop thinking about digital life and nondigital life and just think about life. Parents already know how to parent. What we need to help them do is parent with digital devices and social media with the same good sense they use for all other areas of their children's lives.

TODAY'S FAMILY: DIGITAL USE

Today's family is digital. Knowing the trends of use within a family can assist a health care provider in helping families adjust their use to more age-appropriate limits when necessary.

Parents Today

Parents use of digital media, especially social media, often sets the tone for use within a home. Today's parents are online and are heavy social media users. According to the Pew Research Center, parents use Facebook much more than all other social media platforms followed by Pinterest, LinkedIn, Instagram, and Twitter. With the exception of Twitter, mothers use these platforms more frequently than fathers.[1]

Use by parents is largely informative. Parents use apps and social media to stay connected and up to date. Although documentation via pictures and video is important, it provides a personal goal as opposed to the need to be seen by a wide audience as with their children. Parents "friends" are very personal. Their children's "friends" may not be so.

Parental Concerns

Parents top health concerns have been stable over the last few years, as documented by the CS Mott Children's Hospital National Children's Health Poll. Although the rank order has changed slightly, obesity, bullying, and Internet safety have remained in the top 10 with sexting entering the list most years.[2] These concerns are not surprising because all have a considerable impact on child health, directly and indirectly, and all are related to an ever-growing dependency on digital devices. Obesity, for example, has been linked to children who are heavy game users and digital technology users, in addition to their lack of exercise and poor nutrition. Bullying has an online and offline component. Sexting is a unique online and digital issue that can have lasting consequences. Internet safety has been a stable concern as the digital world has become more prevalent in everyone's lives.

The underlying cause of all concerns related to the digital world, such as those concerning social media use, is a fear from parents that they are in the dark about what their children are doing. Nearly 30% of parents are concerned about technology use in general.[1] The less they know, the more they feel out of touch. This has been occurring at a greater pace as society has become more mobile.

Another major issue is the gap between what parents think their children are doing online and the reality. Parents typically underestimate how much time children are using social media and are not as aware as they think about what they are using for applications.[3] With new applications emerging so quickly, many parents simply cannot keep up and teenagers have learned to be a step ahead of parents by using applications that seem innocent, but are not, and to actually hide what they are doing.

Parents, feeling uncertain, want to lock down technology, but that is not progress for anyone. As with nondigital issues in parenting, helping them foster a forum for communication and parenting with a reasonable approach to the issue at hand produces much better results. This is discussed in more detail later.

Teenage Social Media Use

Teenagers are as digitally tuned in as their parents. Teenage activities fall into distinct groups: communication (texting, messaging), pinboards, gaming, video calls and chats, and photograph documentation. The social media group comprises 15% of all teenagers and tweens.[4]

This is a group that thrives on being involved and their app and social media use centers around these issues. As with their parents, Facebook is the main social media application used, followed by Instagram, Snapchat, Twitter, Google+, and a variety of others. A total of 95% of teenagers 12 and older are online with 80% owning a computer and 77% owning a cellphone.[5] Their digital use is highly mobile with visual apps increasing in use compared with prior surveys, according to Pew Internet.

In addition to the social media applications that their parents use, teenagers gravitate to another group of social media sites that allow for different types of communication. Some of these sites, however, also are also used by young adults and older adults and can be a source for inappropriate contact and cyberbullying. It is important to note these sites and inform parents about them. The more popular sites include Kik, Vine, and YikYak.[6]

POSITIVE ASPECTS OF SOCIAL MEDIA

The positive aspects of social media are well documented. Connection with peers and family, creation of video and pictures, and information gathering are all positive activities, especially for teenagers. Older teenagers and college-age students have also found social media valuable in keeping abreast of activities at school and important safety alerts.[4,7]

Social media is used by middle school and high school students in a variety of ways. Some teachers use social media for assignments. Students use social media to swap homework. School groups use social media to post about activities. Blogs and video creation are also popular activities in these age groups.

THE DARK SIDE OF SOCIAL MEDIA

Social media applications are just tools. Negative situations occur because of misuse of the tool. This may be because a child is too young to use the tool or it is a situation the child is not ready for developmentally. This is no different than when something goes awry from any tool out of the digital sphere. For example, someone trained in electricity would not have the knowledge typically to work with plumbing. A child, for example, would not have the experience to use an electric tool unsupervised or cook in a kitchen until old enough to use the tools in the kitchen and appliances unsupervised. Society goes to great lengths to make sure people have the correct training in technical fields and that children are not in harm's way in their homes when young.

Imbedded in every negative issue is the age of the child. Children are always developing errors of judgment, and vulnerability because of age may increase the chances that some of these situations may occur. At the same time, it is important for parents to understand that one of the most important ways to keep teenagers and younger children safe when using social media is ensure they are the proper age to use it. As with any tool, most mistakes and harm come when using it improperly or at a younger age than it is meant to be used. Would you give a 5 year old the keys to your car? Social media, as with many areas of life, has age-restrictions that are important for parents understand.

Why Age Matters

All social media sites have a minimum age of use, usually age 13. This is set by the Children's Online Privacy Protection Act (COPPA), which protects the information of children younger than 13 from being collected from Web sites and applications. This important Act protects the interests of children too young to negotiate the online world without the supervision of parents.[8] Children 13 and older are teenagers. They have the developmental skills to use sites and applications designed for them, including the faceless communication that these sites embody. This is not simply about stranger danger. This is about everything that comes with a site, such as Facebook, Twitter, Instagram, and YouTube, to name a few of the more popular sites. These sites all have advertisements, content, and posts. Children 13 and older are developmentally ready to understand these concepts and find an adult if something is not appropriate or seems overwhelming. A younger child is not developmentally equipped to negotiate the many paths these sites can take a child down.[7]

To sign up for a typical social media site, a box must be checked that says a person is older than 13. If a child is younger than 13, to get onto a site, that child or the parent must lie about that child's age. If a parent is unsure about whether a social media site complies with COPPA and what the minimum age for having an account is for that site, the parent can check the privacy policy page for that site. The links for the more popular sites are as follows:

Facebook[9]: https://www.facebook.com/help/157793540954833
Instagram[10]: https://help.instagram.com/154475974694511/
Twitter[11]: https://twitter.com/privacy?lang=en
Snapchat[12]: https://www.snapchat.com/terms
Kik[13]: http://www.kik.com/privacy/
Google Sites, including YouTube[14]: https://support.google.com/accounts/answer/1350409?hl=en

The question a parent must ask at this point in the enrollment process is simple: would he or she ever allow that child to lie about his or her age in another setting? For example, would the parent allow the child to lie about his or her age to get into a camp or to get a driver's license or a passport? Typically, the answer to these questions is no. We teach our children to not lie about one's age. This is because we are our age. To lie is to misrepresent who we are. It gives the impression to the people who run the site that the child is able to handle the site and interact with the people on the site.[15]

When we lie about our child's age, and allow our child to lie about his or her age, we also give the message to our child that we can bend some big rules in life when it suits us. Our children remember that and use it again. We lose credibility in our children's eyes.

Safety is important. Our children crawl before they walk and run. They get a learner's permit before a driver's license. They learn to make Jell-O and pudding before baking a cake alone. The digital world is the same way. We should allow them to use age-appropriate apps and games before putting them on social media sites for children older than 13. Everything in its proper time is a lesson that they have to learn.

Parental Mixed Signals

One of the biggest issues in families today is parents who try and place limits on children while overusing technology themselves. The limits have to make sense for what parents are trying to achieve. Punishing a child of any age by taking away technology has never been found to be effective. Instead, a more reasonable family use plan that holds everyone accountable and has parents held to the same rules as adults is the best strategy.[7,15,16]

This concept has been reinforced in society by a variety of "unplugged" campaigns, such as the Sabbath Manifesto's National Day of Unplugging Campaign and Chick-Fil-A unplugged container and the unplugged stacking game.[17,18] All of these campaigns are aimed at helping people become more aware of the need to talk more in their lives and become active in the world without technology. A recent survey of parents by the University of Michigan also drives this concept home by surveying students. The results indicate they want parents to be more present and use technology less.[19] In all the studies the message is clear: parents and children believe the other is too distracted by technology.

Parents Unaware of Online Behavior

Many parents believe they are aware of their children's and teenagers' online activities. However, studies continue to confirm that children and teenagers are savvy at hiding their online activities. This is particularly true for social media. A 2012 study by McAfee showed that although 49% of parents surveyed installed some sort of control, 71% of teenagers did something to hide their online behavior with only 56% of parents aware.[3] For example, according to the study, 53.3% of teenagers "clear browser history" with 17.5% parents aware, 22.9% of teenagers lied about behavior with 10.5% parents aware, and 19.9% teenagers manipulated social media privacy settings to block parents with 8.1% parents aware. There were also many teenagers with duplicate email addresses, with many parents unaware. A more recent study has shown that 44% of children and teenagers hide their information from parents.[20]

iPhone Thumb

This condition emerged with the popularity of hand-held devices and gaming systems and has gone through several name changes. Initially known as "Nintendo-itis," today it is best known as iPhone thumb and is an overuse phenomenon of the hands and wrists. With the rise of smartphones and texting, the fingers and thumbs have become especially susceptible.

Patients usually complain of pain, swelling, and decreased range of motion in the affected area. Sometimes there may be redness and warmth. Treatment is supportive with rest, reducing the amount of time with the offending activity, ice, and nonsteroidal anti-inflammatory agents.[21]

Back and Neck Problems

Hands are not the only part of the body impacted by technology use. Researchers and clinicians have long observed people complaining of back and neck straining as technology has consumed greater proportions of our lives. The more people have complained, the more researchers have taken an interest in these issues. Recently, researchers have noted that as people have become more mobile, their posture has changed, looking down more and changing how we hold our spines. This has created a great force on the neck, shoulders, and spine.[22] A study out of New York Spine Surgery revealed that adults can spend 2 to 4 hours looking down, which amounts to 700 to 1400 hours a year. This research group estimates that high school students may extend this amount by 5000 hours. These researchers postulate that the longer everyone stays in these abnormal positions, the more we are all at risk for cervical scoliosis and breakdown of cervical tissues. The concern is not academic. There could be the need for surgery if the dysfunction becomes great enough over time.

The solution to this problem is uncertain. However, with experience from other technologies and health, it is known that balance and moderation are always part of a good lifestyle. Teaching our children to take breaks from technology goes a long way in breaking bad habits. We can be good role models. One good practice is to balance hand-held devices with computer use, take stretching breaks, and use tablets mixed with phones.

Social Media Distractions

Distractions from social media are becoming a new health issues as mobile technology has become a larger part of every generation's digital lives. As a result, injuries from using mobile technology while doing routine activities, such as driving, walking, or even biking, are starting to become a bigger concern.

Driving

One of the most dangerous activities while driving is texting. Studies have found that texting while driving distracts a driver in such way that his or her impairment is worse than if impaired by alcohol.[23] One of the earliest studies done by Car and Driver compared texting and reading with being intoxicated by alcohol as defined by legal breathalyzer limits. Both texting and reading were found to impair a driver worse than alcohol intoxication.

Most states now have legal remedies to deal with this dangerous issue. A total of 46 states now have bans on texting while driving for all drivers, with 38 states banning texting for novice drivers.[24]

Walking

Walking with a mobile device, especially while trying to text or use another app, is as dangerous as driving while texting. SafeKids reports that one in five high school students and one in eight middle school students is distracted while crossing the street.[25] Emergency room visits for accidents to people using phones while walking are steadily increasing with more than 1500 visits reported in 2010. This is a doubling in injuries over the last decade.[26]

Body Image and Self-Esteem

Social media is a huge shaper of body image today, especially in teenage girls. It acts as a mirror for comparison and can have a positive and negative impact. Social media can impact self-esteem positively and negatively depending on how a picture of a girl is received online.[4] Educating teenagers about the impact of social media in general, and specifically on body image, and being aware of body image issues in a teenager is how to help parents with this issue.

Digital Dangers: Cyberbully, Sexting, and Inappropriate Content

Digital dangers, such as cyberbullying, sexting, and accessing inappropriate content, are well documented in other reports.[7] They are common dangers with any social media use and something parents need to be aware about. However, studies continue to document that parents underestimate that their teenagers can get into trouble online at all, let alone by these significant dangers. McAfee reports that only 21% of parents believe their children are at risk of danger online.[3]

These are concerns that parents have annually.[2] There is a disconnect in parents thinking about the digital lives of their children. For them to understand their link to social media, the first step is helping them understand the data on how many children are impacted by each issue.

SUMMARY

Parents seek information on problems they fear are impacting their children's lives. Technology, however, is impacting the entire family. Parents, too, are affected with the same issues as their children. Parents use and overuse social media. Parents are distracted at home, while walking, and while driving. Parental engagement with others has decreased as society has become more about digital connections and less about social connections. The solution for parents to help their children with technology and gain more control over everyone's digital lives is to unplug more, and regain true family connections.

As health care providers, it is important to help allay parental concerns about social media. To do so, adding pertinent digital parenting advice, especially about social media, to all health care visits is a necessary first step. In addition, the following recommendations may assist in helping parents as they work to keep their children safe and healthy in today's evolving world:

1. Reinforce to parents that they already have the parenting skills they need to parent a digital child. Parenting a digital issue requires the same skills as a nondigital issue. The first step is knowledge about that issue followed by a reasonable approach for that problem.
2. Help parents recognize that one of the most powerful ways to help children in every issue today is to be a good role model. For social media, moderating their own use, practicing good social media habits, and being away from their devices when true social connections with family and friends are needed are the starting points.
3. Help parents know the privacy rules and about COPPA. Parents should understand that if it is not acceptable to break a law offline, it is not acceptable online. The digital world now has laws that apply to its use. For children and teenagers to understand those laws, parents need to as well, and need to follow those laws. If parents keep crossing those lines, children will, too.
4. A family digital use plan is one of the best ways to help parents and children of all ages follow the appropriate rules. Have one available to hand out for your families to use as a starting point.
5. Inform your families that you are available to help for digital issues, such as cyberbullying and sexting. If they know these tough issues are today's new health issues, they will call you if an issue arises.

The collective goal is to help families achieve a happy medium from a place of understanding, not fear. As they reconnect, they will find that place, especially if we help them get there.

REFERENCES

1. Duggan M, Lenhart A, Lampe C, et al. Parents and social media. Pew Research Center; 2015. Available at: http://www.pewinternet.org/2015/07/16/parents-and-social-media/. Accessed April 18, 2016.
2. Top 10 U.S. children's health concerns in 2015. Ann Arbor, MI: C.S.Mott Children's Hospital; 2015. Available at: http://mottnpch.org/blog/2015-08-18/top-10-us-childrens-health-concerns-2015. Accessed March 15, 2016.
3. The digital divide: how the online behavior of teens is getting past parents (n.d.): n. page. 1 2012. Available at: http://www.mcafee.com/us/about/news/2012/q2/20120625-01.aspx. Accessed March 16, 2016.
4. Rideout V. The common sense census: media use by tweens and teens. San Francisco, CA: Common Sense Media Research; 2015. Available at: https://www.commonsensemedia.org/research/the-common-sense-census-media-use-by-tweens-and-teens. Accessed March 21, 2016.
5. Lenhart A, Smith A, Anderson M. Teens, technology and romantic relationships. Washington, DC: Pew Research Center; 2015. Available at: http://www.pewinternet.org/2015/10/01/teens-technology-and-romantic-relationships/10. Accessed March 15, 2016.
6. Elgersma C. 16 apps and websites kids are heading to after Facebook. Reviews & age ratings. San Francisco, CA: Common Sense Media; 2016. Available at: https://www.commonsensemedia.org/blog/16-apps-and-websites-kids-are-heading-to-after-facebook. Accessed April 18, 2016.
7. O'Keeffe GS, Clarke-Pearson K. The impact of social media on children, adolescents, and families. Pediatrics 2011;127(4):800–4.
8. Complying with COPPA: frequently asked questions. Federal Trade Commission. Washington, DC: Federal Trade Commission; 2015. Available at: https://www.ftc.gov/tips-advice/business-center/guidance/complying-coppa-frequently-asked-questions25. Accessed April 18, 2016.
9. Facebook. How do I report a child under the age of 13? Facebook, n.d. Available at: https://www.facebook.com/help/157793540954833. Accessed April 18, 2016.
10. Instagram Help Center. Tips for parents. Instagram, n.d. Available at: https://help.instagram.com/154475974694511/. Accessed April 18, 2016.
11. Twitter Privacy Policy. Twitter. Twitter, n.d. Available at: https://twitter.com/privacy?lang=en. Accessed April 18, 2016.
12. Terms of Service. Snapchat. Snapchat. 2016. Available at: https://www.snapchat.com/terms. Accessed April 18, 2016.
13. Privacy Policy. Privacy » Kik. Kik, n.d. Available at: https://www.kik.com/privacy/. Accessed April 18, 2016.
14. Age Requirements on Google Accounts. Accounts Help. Google, n.d. Available at: https://support.google.com/accounts/answer/1350409?hl=en. Accessed April 18, 2016.
15. O'Keeffe GS. CyberSafe. Elk Grove Village, IL: AAP Books; 2005. p. 247–9, 179–182.
16. National Day of Unplugging - March 7th, 2014. Sabbath Manifesto. National Day of Unplugging. 2017. Available at: http://nationaldayofunplugging.com. Accessed April 18, 2016.

17. Ward S. How putting the phone down for dinner became a family challenge. Available at: http://www.today.com/food/chick-fil-s-cell-phone-coop-other-eateries-encourage-diners-t77226. Accessed June 20, 2016.
18. Inside ChickfilA. Chick-fil-A. 2016. Avaialble at: http://inside.chick-fil-a.com/all-cooped-up-how-one-chick-fil-a-operator-is-redefining-the-phrase/. Accessed April 18, 2016.
19. Family technology rules: what kids expect of parents. Ann Arbor, MI: School of Information. University of Michigan; 2016. Available at: https://www.si.umich.edu/news/family-technology-rules-what-kids-expect-parents28. Accessed April 18, 2016.
20. Kaspersky lab study finds half of children hide risky online behavior from parents. Woburn, MA: Kaspersky Labs; 2016. Available at: http://usa.kaspersky.com/about-us/press-center/press-releases/2016/Kaspersky-Lab-Study-Finds-Half-of-Children-Hide-Risky-Online-Behavior-from-Parents. Accessed April 18, 2016.
21. Smartphone thumb: when the toys we love don't love us back - Orthopedics, Spine & Sports Medicine. Atlanta, GA: Orthopedics Spine Sports Medicine. Emory Healthcare; 2012. Available at: http://advancingyourhealth.org/orthopedics/2012/05/11/what-is-smartphone-thumb-prevention/. Accessed April 18, 2016.
22. Hansraj KK. Assessment of stresses in the cervical spine caused by posture and position of the head. Surg Technol Int 2014;25:277–9.
23. Austin M. Texting while driving: how dangerous is it? - Feature. Car and Driver. N.p. 2009. Avaialble at: http://inside.chick-fil-a.com/all-cooped-up-how-one-chick-fil-a-operator-is-redefining-the-phrase/. Accessed April 8, 2016.
24. State Laws. Distracted driving. Available at: Distraction.Gov. Accessed April 18, 2016.
25. Pedestrian Fatalities. Encyclopedia of trauma care (2015): 18. Elk Grove Village, IL: Governor's Highway Safety Association; 2016. Available at: http://www.ghsa.org/html/publications/spotlight/peds2015.html. Accessed April 18, 2016.
26. Research and Innovation Communications. Distracted walking: injuries soar for pedestrians on phones. Columbus, OH: The Ohio State University; 2013. Available at: http://researchnews.osu.edu/archive/distractwalk.htm. Accessed April 18, 2016.

Whittling Down the Wait Time

Exploring Models to Minimize the Delay from Initial Concern to Diagnosis and Treatment of Autism Spectrum Disorder

Eliza Gordon-Lipkin, MD[a],*, Jessica Foster, MD, MPH[b], Georgina Peacock, MD, MPH[c]

KEYWORDS

- Autism spectrum disorder • Diagnosis • Wait-list • Children

KEY POINTS

- The "diagnostic odyssey" in autism, from initial concerns to diagnosis, is often a long and complicated process for families, prolonged by wait-lists due to a backlog of patients awaiting evaluation by subspecialists.
- Multiple clinical autism centers throughout the United States have implemented innovative programs to directly address this diagnostic bottleneck, resulting in decreased wait times in their local communities.
- A change in clinical approach from a focus on diagnosis to a focus on referral to therapeutic services may better serve families as they undergo diagnostic evaluation.
- A public health approach that intersects with clinical care is needed to facilitate diagnosis and acquisition of services for children with autism.

Over the last several decades, autism spectrum disorder (ASD) has become an increasingly recognized developmental disability, affecting thousands of children, adults, and their families. According to the most recent statistics,[1] 1 in 68 school-aged children in the United States has been identified with ASD. This prevalence

The authors have nothing to disclose.
The findings and conclusions in this report are those of the authors and do not necessarily represent the official position of the Centers for Disease Control and Prevention.
[a] Department of Neurology and Developmental Medicine, Kennedy Krieger Institute, 716 North Broadway, Baltimore, MD 21205, USA; [b] Section of Developmental Pediatrics, Akron Children's Hospital, Neuro Developmental Science Center, Considine Professional Building, 215 West Bowery Street, Suite 4400, Akron, OH 44308, USA; [c] Division of Human Development and Disability, National Center on Birth Defects and Developmental Disabilities, Centers for Disease Control and Prevention, 4770 Buford Hwy MS-E88, Atlanta, GA 30329, USA
* Corresponding author. Kennedy Krieger Institute, 716 North Broadway, Baltimore, MD 21205.
E-mail address: lipkinE@kennedykrieger.org

Pediatr Clin N Am 63 (2016) 851–859
http://dx.doi.org/10.1016/j.pcl.2016.06.007   pediatric.theclinics.com
0031-3955/16/$ – see front matter © 2016 Elsevier Inc. All rights reserved.

has increased over the last decade, from 1 in 150 in 2002, to 1 in 110 in 2006, to 1 in 68 in 2010[2] and 2012.[1,3–5]

Children with ASD can be diagnosed as early as 2 years of age,[6,7] but on average, the age of diagnosis is after 4 years.[2] There is even evidence that parents may detect developmental concerns in children with ASD before 12 months of age.[8,9] There are multiple factors that account for the more than the 2-year difference between earliest signs to diagnosis that may delay entry into early intervention (EI) programs. These barriers, which include time-consuming evaluations,[10] cost of care,[11] lack of providers,[12] lack of comfort in diagnosing by primary care providers,[12] and other challenges, each require different approaches in order to begin to close this gap.

There is also increasing emphasis on earlier identification of ASD and initiation of specialized interventions, due to evidence that starting these therapies as early as 18 months leads to better long-term outcomes.[13–15] The American Academy of Pediatrics (AAP) and other professional organizations have therefore emphasized that children with suspected or confirmed ASD should receive services that address a combination of approaches, and that therapy should begin as soon as possible.[16]

As such, ASD as an increasing public health concern has not gone unnoticed. Multiple legislative efforts have been made to support ASD awareness and services. ASD is included as a diagnosis of eligibility under the Individuals with Disabilities Education Act, established in 1990 to provide EI therapeutic services to children under age 3 years with disabilities. The US Congress later passed the Combating Autism Act of 2006, followed by the Autism Care Act in 2014, funding ASD research, surveillance, and education. The Centers for Disease Control and Prevention has also held collaborative summits in an effort to support states' abilities to implement early identification programs and EI services for children with ASD.[17] Often these EI services are supplemented with additional therapies. Insurance coverage is variable across therapy type and can be quite different in different states. Having an ASD diagnosis can change the type and amount of coverage that a child may have through insurance and public EI and education programs.

These collaborative efforts have yielded research and screening tools to detect ASD signs and symptoms in children less than 24 months of age.[18] Despite this, mean age of diagnosis in the United States remains stable at 3.5 to 5 years.[1,2] Multiple factors influence the process described by parents as the "diagnostic odyssey," from first concerns to age of diagnosis. Most notably, throughout the country, there is a backlog of patients waiting to be seen[11] and a lack of qualified providers.[19]

Thus, there exists a need for a public health approach that intersects with clinical care in order to facilitate diagnosis and acquisition of services for children with ASD. In this article, the authors describe the traditional models for this process as well as new and innovative approaches to address this issue.

THE AUTISM "DIAGNOSTIC ODYSSEY": THE TRADITIONAL MODEL

For most families, initial concerns for ASD are brought up by a parent at a routine well-child visit or identified by routine screening at the 18- and 24-month well-child visit.[20] Ideally, according to AAP guidelines, a child is then referred by the provider for audiologic evaluation, EI education services, and a comprehensive ASD evaluation.

Therefore, what is a comprehensive ASD evaluation? There is wide variability in the clinical structure of these subspecialty service providers[21]; however, in many clinical settings, a comprehensive ASD evaluation consists of a visit or multiple visits for evaluations by a multidisciplinary team, including a physician, psychologist, speech language pathologist, and sometimes other providers, such as a social worker, occupational therapist, and/or genetic counselor. Each specialist brings different expertise to aid in diagnosis and recommendations for the patient. These comprehensive assessments include clinical evaluation as well as use of standardized instruments. The ADOS,[22] or Autism Diagnostic Observation Schedule, has become the gold-standard diagnostic tool and is often helpful, but not required, for a diagnosis of ASD. The ADOS is a 40- to 60-minute, play-based, standardized assessment for children 12 months and up that is typically performed by a developmental pediatrician, speech language pathologist, or psychologist. This evaluation, as well as other neuropsychological testing and medical evaluation by a developmental pediatrician, child neurologist, or child psychiatrist, is taken to provide a comprehensive diagnosis and recommendations for therapeutic services.

This multidisciplinary team approach can provide excellent comprehensive evaluation, diagnosis, and detailed recommendations. However, these evaluations are time-consuming for both the patient and the care team. Some clinics require a screening process before scheduling appointments with forms of up to 200 questions.[11] Clinical testing can take 2 to 3 hours in addition to face-to-face time spent with the physician, and some clinics require more than 3 separate visits.[21] Consequently, clinics are limited in the number of patients that can be seen.

In addition, there exist national shortages of subspecialist providers, adding to the wait time for diagnosis. A 2012 survey by the Children's Hospital Association reported national shortages in all of the pediatric subspecialties that diagnose and treat ASD: Developmental Pediatrics, Pediatric Neurology, and Child and Adolescent Psychiatry.[23] According to this study and others, the average wait time to schedule an appointment with these specialists was 3.5 months[11]; however, in some areas of the country, wait times are significantly longer, and it may take up to a year to have a comprehensive evaluation.[24] Families are highly dependent on resources in their local community, which may be variable. In rural settings, access to subspecialists for ASD evaluation is even more difficult, as most multidisciplinary teams practice in major urban academic centers. Only 7% of developmental pediatricians practice in rural areas. Some states do not have a developmental pediatrician.[25]

Ideally, toddlers suspected of having ASD are referred to Part C EI services at the same time that concerns arise, and they are enrolled in services as they await a subspecialty evaluation. A diagnosis of ASD is not required to qualify for these EI services. However, in many cases, children are not referred to EI services until *after* a confirmed diagnosis that results from a comprehensive ASD evaluation, which may be many months later. Once a child has a diagnosis of ASD as opposed to nonspecific developmental delay, the type of services he or she receives may change. An ASD diagnosis may allow the child to be eligible for different and increased services, specific to ASD. These services often include ABA or applied behavioral analysis therapy, an evidence-based technique that has proven efficacy in ASD.[26–28]

NOVEL AND INNOVATIVE MODELS FOR AUTISM SPECTRUM DISORDER DIAGNOSIS

The problem of prolonged wait times for ASD diagnosis and services has not gone unrecognized by families or by ASD service providers. Public outcry has spurred multiple autism centers around the country to devise creative and novel clinical models to reduce the waiting time that families endure between initial concerns and diagnosis, delaying initiation of therapy.

Autism Diagnosis Education Project

In Ohio, the substantial wait times experienced at specialty autism centers and the lag time from initial concern to diagnosis of ASD sparked the development of the Autism Diagnosis Education Project (ADEP).[22] ADEP was developed in collaboration with ASD providers and leaders in state public health and early childhood education. ADEP facilitates unique partnerships between community-based primary care practices and professionals providing EI and early childhood services, to increase access to local and timely standardized, comprehensive diagnostic evaluations for children suspected of having an ASD. Launched in 2008, the ADEP was originally piloted through funds from the Ohio Department of Health and administered by the Ohio Chapter of the AAP. The piloting of the project concluded in June 2011. The ADEP resumed and was expanded in October 2012 with funding from the Governor's Office of Health Transformation, awarded to the Ohio Department of Developmental Disabilities. The Department partnered with Akron Children's Hospital, Family Child Learning Center, and the Ohio Center for Autism and Low Incidence to coordinate and implement the ADEP expansion. The project's work aligns with the Ohio Autism Recommendations,[29] which emphasizes the importance of early identification and diagnosis of autism.

The goals of the expanded ADEP included (1) reduction of the time from initial family concern to diagnosis from 18 months to less than 9 months; (2) reduction of the time from initial contact with Ohio's Help Me Grow[30] assessment system to diagnosis to within 90 days; and (3) lowering the age of diagnosis from age 36 months to 30 months. Through persistent efforts and a willingness to overcome barriers, the teams involved with ADEP have lowered the average age of diagnosis in Ohio to 28.9 months of age.[29] This age is still above the age of 24 months, which has been found to be an age at which autism diagnosis remains stable. The ADEP teams continue to change the ways in which families can receive an early diagnosis of ASD in the state of Ohio.

Vanderbilt Treatment and Research Institute for Autism Spectrum Disorders

Vanderbilt Treatment and Research Institute for Autism Spectrum Disorders (TRIAD) developed a program[31–33] specifically to address the underserved areas in the state of Tennessee, where wait times for diagnostic or interventional services for children with ASD can be as long as 6 to 12 months. They advocate training primary care practitioners to use a validated interactive screening tool for ASD called STAT (Screening Tool for Autism in Toddlers and Young Children).[31,32] The STAT is an approximately 20-minute assessment that evaluates toddlers ages 24 to 35 months using 12 interactive items based on social-communication behaviors evidenced to differentiate 2 year olds with and without ASD. This measure has been validated to correctly identify 75% to 90% of children with ASD.

In their model, the Vanderbilt team suggests that children with a positive ASD screen at routine 18- and 24-month pediatric visits could then undergo the STAT as a prompt diagnostic assessment within primary care providers' clinical practices. The Vanderbilt team has initiated training programs in order to develop a network of pediatricians throughout the state who are capable of identifying and immediately referring children at high risk for ASD for appropriate EI services, avoiding long waits for diagnosis or treatment.[34,35] On follow-up, this network of primary care pediatricians reported an 85% increase in diagnosis of children with ASD within their own practices. Extrapolating to address the statewide need for ASD evaluation services in Tennessee, it was estimated that 20 pediatricians performing one assessment per week could serve more than 1000 patients a year.[36]

Community-based Autism Liaison and Treatment Program

Several other states have developed similar programs that train local pediatricians to diagnose ASD. Arkansas has created the Community-based Autism Liaison and Treatment, or CoBALT Program, an educational training program for "mini-teams" of one community-based pediatrician coupled with a one speech language patholo-gist. The goal of this training is to establish community-based teams capable of providing diagnostic developmental assessments. The CoBALT program also empha-sizes directly connecting these trainees to representatives in the local EI, Early Child-hood Special Education, and Department of Developmental Services programs, and other services in order to facilitate network building and communication within the pro-fessional community that serves these children.[37] Since its start in 2011, the CoBALT program has trained 12 teams that provide services throughout the state of Arkansas, including rural counties.

Other centers around the country are starting to develop their own creative models to tackle this same problem. Connecticut Children's Medical Center has an Autism Spectrum Assessment Program that reports to have reduced wait times by half.[38] Their model focuses on obtaining comprehensive information before the appointment, simultaneously referring to EI and capitalizing on the increased ratio of speech lan-guage pathologists to developmental pediatricians by using the physicians on an as needed basis.[39]

A second program in Ohio focuses on reducing wait times within their own ASD intervention centers at Cincinnati Children's Hospital Medical Center and Nationwide Children's Hospital by systemic analysis of supply, demand, and activity to identify and target sources of delay.[24] Their analysis found that by collapsing multiple visit types and reducing the complexity within the clinical system, as well as reviewing wait lists and modifying wait list policies in favor of scheduling more appointments, these centers successfully reduced the wait time and nearly eliminated wait lists.

ADDITIONAL OPPORTUNITIES IN TECHNOLOGY AND PUBLIC POLICY

Other opportunities may exist for creative models that improve access to care for chil-dren requiring evaluation for ASD. Some of these next steps capitalize on modern technology or may call for changes in public policy. Here, a few examples of models that have the potential to further expand upon the strategies above are discussed.

Telemedicine programs are expanding throughout medicine, including those that focus on developmental disabilities, and have improved access to care, particularly for patients in rural settings.[40] There is emerging research on applying this practice for children with ASD in a variety of ways. Some centers have published studies reporting that ASD evaluations performed through video conferences directly between a family and an interdisciplinary team may be an accurate and accessible means for evaluation.[41–44] Other centers have used telemedicine to provide peer-to-peer sub-specialty consultations[45,46] for developmental disabilities, in their local communities and internationally.[47] One study has even designed a diagnostic tool using home videos recorded by parents.[48] Specifically, a program in Kansas uses professional teams in the patient's local community to perform standardized assessments, which are then presented to the family and a university-based medical center team that makes the final diagnostic assessment and provides recommendations via telemedi-cine.[42] As academic hospital centers rapidly expand their technological resources, telemedicine provides a modern venue for increasing accessibility to specialized ser-vices for children with developmental concerns.

Additional efforts that have been considered directly address the shortage of pediatric subspecialty providers, including those that provide services for children with ASD: developmental pediatricians, child neurologists, and child and adolescent psychiatrists. The AAP has issued a policy statement[19] delineating objectives to increase the numbers of appropriately trained pediatric subspecialists. They have also advocated for legislation that provides incentives for new physicians to pursue pediatric subspecialties through graduate medical education funding, loan repayment programs, training grants, and appropriate payment for services.[49] Specifically, legislation being considered by Congress includes the Ensuring Children's Access to Specialty Care Act of 2015 (H.R. 1859) that would amend the Public Health Service Act to include pediatric subspecialists in the National Health Service Corps loan repayment program. In addition, the House and Senate Labor-Health and Human Services-Education appropriations bills authorized funding for the Children's Hospital Graduate Medical Education program, which provides funding to support pediatric residency and fellowship positions.[50]

Finally, it has been suggested that the development of open source and open access tools to diagnose for autism may eliminate some of barriers in the diagnostic process.[51] Currently, the high costs to use these proprietary tools and to train professionals to use them consequently limit the number of proficient providers, particularly in resources-limited settings, and may add to the bottleneck for families at ASD centers. In contrast to many of the "gold-standard" assessments such as the ADOS[22] and Autism Diagnostic Interview–Revised,[52] open source tools are free to access without cost. Introducing more open access diagnostic tools may have the potential to facilitate the ASD diagnostic process, particularly in low-resource settings.

NEXT STEPS

All of the novel models discussed have shown positive impact on the local communities that they serve. However, efforts to redesign clinical services for the diagnosis of ASD are not pervasive in the medical community. This lack of generalized reform of clinical models is evidenced by the fact that despite substantial efforts by these and other programs, the average age of ASD diagnosis in the United States has still not declined. There is still more work to do to implement innovative programs on a national scale.

In general, many of these approaches focus on simultaneously referring children for services while the diagnostic process is underway. This multifaceted strategy of simultaneous referral and diagnostic workup underscores a need for a change in the clinical approach to ASD from a primary focus of diagnostic labeling to a focus on function. A functional approach[53] may better serve the child and the family by prioritizing implementation of services and therapies as soon as concerns are identified in order to improve the outcome for that child. Limiting these services based on a diagnostic label may only detrimentally delay this process.

The diagnostic odyssey for parents of children with ASD remains a challenging process that demands remodeling from the clinician level to the public health level in order to better serve families. Some promising ideas are emerging to address these needs. The systems of care built to identify ASD need to continue to evolve in order to serve the growing number of individuals with ASD that await their services.

REFERENCES

1. Christensen DL, Jon B, Van Naarden Braun K, et al. Prevalence and characteristics of autism spectrum disorder among children aged 8 years—autism and

developmental disabilities monitoring network, 11 sites, United States, 2012. MMWR Surveill Summ 2016;65(3):1–23.

2. Developmental Disabilities Monitoring Network Surveillance Year 2010 Principal Investigators, Centers for Disease Control and Prevention (CDC). Prevalence of autism spectrum disorder among children aged 8 years—autism and developmental disabilities monitoring network, 11 sites, United States, 2010. MMWR Surveill Summ 2014;63(2):1–21.

3. Christensen DL, Bilder DA, Zahorodny W, et al. Prevalence and characteristics of autism spectrum disorder among 4-year-old children in the autism and developmental disabilities monitoring network. J Dev Behav Pediatr 2016;37(1):1–8.

4. Zablotsky B, Black LI, Maenner MJ, et al. Estimated prevalence of autism and other developmental disabilities following questionnaire changes in the 2014 National Health Interview Survey. Natl Health Stat Rep 2015;(87):1–20.

5. Mack AH. Prevalence of autism spectrum disorders—autism and developmental disabilities monitoring network, United States, 2006. Year Bk Psychiatr Appl Ment Health 2011;2011:37–9.

6. Kleinman JM, Ventola PE, Pandey J, et al. Diagnostic stability in very young children with autism spectrum disorders. J Autism Dev Disord 2008;38(4):606–15.

7. Lord C, Risi S, DiLavore PS, et al. Autism from 2 to 9 years of age. Arch Gen Psychiatry 2006;63(6):694–701.

8. Kozlowski AM, Matson JL, Max H, et al. Parents' first concerns of their child's development in toddlers with autism spectrum disorders. Dev Neurorehabil 2011;14(2):72–8.

9. Bolton PF, Golding J, Emond A, et al. Autism spectrum disorder and autistic traits in the Avon Longitudinal Study of Parents and Children: precursors and early signs. J Am Acad Child Adolesc Psychiatry 2012;51(3):249–60.e25.

10. Kalb LG, Freedman B, Foster C, et al. Determinants of appointment absenteeism at an outpatient pediatric autism clinic. J Dev Behav Pediatr 2012;33(9):685–97.

11. Bisgaier J, Levinson D, Cutts DB, et al. Access to autism evaluation appointments with developmental-behavioral and neurodevelopmental subspecialists. Arch Pediatr Adolesc Med 2011;165(7):673–4.

12. Fenikile TS, Sunny Fenikile T, Kathryn E, et al. Barriers to autism screening in family medicine practice: a qualitative study. J Dev Behav Pediatr 2010; 31(Abstracts):E15–6.

13. Estes A, Munson J, Rogers SJ, et al. Long-term outcomes of early intervention in 6-year-old children with autism spectrum disorder. J Am Acad Child Adolesc Psychiatry 2015;54(7):580–7.

14. Remington B, Bob R, Hastings RP, et al. Early intensive behavioral intervention: outcomes for children with autism and their parents after two years. Am J Ment Retard 2007;112(6):418.

15. Dawson G, Rogers S, Munson J, et al. Randomized, controlled trial of an intervention for toddlers with autism: the Early Start Denver Model. Pediatrics 2010; 125(1):e17–23.

16. Zwaigenbaum L, Bauman ML, Choueiri R, et al. Early intervention for children with autism spectrum disorder under 3 years of age: recommendations for practice and research. Pediatrics 2015;136(Suppl 1):S60–81.

17. Peacock G, Lin SC. Enhancing early identification and coordination of intervention services for young children with autism spectrum disorders: report from the Act Early Regional Summit Project. Disabil Health J 2012;5(1):55–9.

18. Sacrey L-AR, Bennett JA, Zwaigenbaum L. Early infant development and intervention for autism spectrum disorder. J Child Neurol 2015;30(14):1921–9.

19. Basco WT, Rimsza ME, Committee on Pediatric Workforce. Pediatrician workforce policy statement. Pediatrics 2013;132(2):390–7.
20. Johnson CP, Myers SM, American Academy of Pediatrics Council on Children With Disabilities. Identification and evaluation of children with autism spectrum disorders. Pediatrics 2007;120(5):1183–215.
21. Hansen RL, Blum NJ, Gaham A, et al. Diagnosis of autism spectrum disorder by developmental-behavioral pediatricians in academic centers: a DBPNet Study. Pediatrics 2016;137(Suppl 2):S79–89.
22. Le Couteur A, Rutter M, Lord C, et al. Autism diagnostic interview: a standardized investigator-based instrument. J Autism Dev Disord 1989;19(3):363–87.
23. Pediatric Specialist Physician Shortages Affect Access to Care. Available at: https://www.childrenshospitals.org/~/media/Files/CHA/Main/Issues_and_Advocacy/Key_Issues/Graduate_Medical_Education/Fact_Sheets/Pediatric_Specialist_Physician_Shortages_Affect_Access_to_Care08012012.pdf. Accessed March 1, 2016.
24. Austin J, Manning-Courtney P, Johnson ML, et al. Improving access to care at autism treatment centers: a system analysis approach. Pediatrics 2016; 137(Suppl 2):S149–57.
25. Althouse LA, Stockman JA 3rd. Pediatric workforce: a look at pediatric nephrology data from the American Board of Pediatrics. J Pediatr 2006;148(5): 575–6.
26. Smith T, Iadarola S. Evidence base update for autism spectrum disorder. J Clin Child Adolesc Psychol 2015;44(6):897–922.
27. Spreckley M, Boyd R. Efficacy of applied behavioral intervention in preschool children with autism for improving cognitive, language, and adaptive behavior: a systematic review and meta-analysis. J Pediatr 2009;154(3):338–44.
28. Sallows GO, Graupner TD. Intensive behavioral treatment for children with autism: four-year outcome and predictors. Am J Ment Retard 2005;110(6): 417–38.
29. OCALI. Ohio ADEP Expansion Report. 2015.
30. Ohio Department of Health: Help Me Grow. Ohio.gov. Available at: http://www.helpmegrow.ohio.gov/. Accessed April 4, 2016.
31. Stone WL, Coonrod EE, Turner LM, et al. Psychometric properties of the STAT for early autism screening. J Autism Dev Disord 2004;34(6):691–701.
32. Stone WL. Screening tool for autism in two-year-olds (STAT). Encyclopedia of autism spectrum disorders. 2013. p. 2684–2688.
33. Humberd Q, Stone W, Warren Z. STAT-MD training. Vanderbilt Kennedy Center. Available at: http://vkc.mc.vanderbilt.edu/vkc/triad/training/stat/physicians/. Accessed April 4, 2016.
34. Swanson AR, Warren ZE, Stone WL, et al. The diagnosis of autism in community pediatric settings: Does advanced training facilitate practice change? Autism 2013;18(5):555–61.
35. Kobak KA, Stone WL, Ousley OY, et al. Web-based training in early autism screening: results from a pilot study. Telemed J E Health 2011;17(8):640–4.
36. Warren Z, Stone W, Humberd Q. A training model for the diagnosis of autism in community pediatric practice. J Dev Behav Pediatr 2009;30(5):442–6.
37. Schulz E. Executive summary: capacity building for ASD and DD: Community-Based Autism Liaison and Training (CoBALT) Project in Arkansas. 2016.
38. Autism Spectrum Assessment Program. Connecticut Children's Medical Center. Available at: http://www.connecticutchildrens.org/our-care/developmental-and-rehabilitation-medicine/programs-services/autism-spectrum-assessment-program/. Accessed April 3, 2016.

39. Twachtman-Bassett J. Filling a need to reduce wait time for Autism assessments: the Autism Spectrum Assessment Program at Connecticut Children's Medical Center. Available at: http://www.amchp.org/programsandtopics/CYSHCN/projects/spharc/peer-to-peer-exchange/Documents/Filling-a-need-Reduce-Wait-Time-Slides.pdf. Accessed April 4, 2016.
40. Marcin JP, Shaikh U, Steinhorn RH. Addressing health disparities in rural communities using telehealth. Pediatr Res 2016;79(1–2):169–76.
41. Reese RM, Jamison TR, Braun M, et al. Brief report: use of interactive television in identifying autism in young children: methodology and preliminary data. J Autism Dev Disord 2015;45(5):1474–82.
42. Reese RM, Braun MJ, Hoffmeier S, et al. Preliminary evidence for the integrated systems using telemedicine. Telemed J E Health 2015;21(7):581–7.
43. Schutte JL, McCue MP, Parmanto B, et al. Usability and reliability of a remotely administered adult autism assessment, the autism diagnostic observation schedule (ADOS) module 4. Telemed J E Health 2015;21(3):176–84.
44. Reese RM, Jamison R, Wendland M, et al. Evaluating interactive videoconferencing for assessing symptoms of autism. Telemed J E Health 2013;19(9):671–7.
45. Arora S, Sanjeev A, Karla T, et al. Outcomes of treatment for hepatitis C virus infection by primary care providers. N Engl J Med 2011;364(23):2199–207.
46. Show-Me ECHO: Missouri Telehealth Network. Available at: www.showmeecho.com. Accessed April 4, 2016.
47. Pearl PL, Sable C, Evans S, et al. International telemedicine consultations for neurodevelopmental disabilities. Telemed J E Health 2014;20(6):559–62.
48. Nazneen N, Rozga A, Smith CJ, et al. A novel system for supporting autism diagnosis using home videos: iterative development and evaluation of system design. JMIR Mhealth Uhealth 2015;3(2):e68.
49. Baumberger JD, Jorgensen-Earp E. Washington Report: Academic and Subspecialty Advocacy. American Academy of Pediatrics. Available at: http://downloads.aap.org/DOSP/SubspecialtyAdvocacy-Oct2015.pdf. Accessed April 4, 2016.
50. One Hundred Ninth Congress of the United States of America. Children's Hospital GME Support Reauthorization Act of 2006. 2006. Available at: https://www.gpo.gov/fdsys/pkg/BILLS-109hr5574enr/pdf/BILLS-109hr5574enr.pdf.
51. Durkin MS, Elsabbagh M, Barbaro J, et al. Autism screening and diagnosis in low resource settings: Challenges and opportunities to enhance research and services worldwide. Autism Res 2015;8(5):473–6.
52. Lord C, Rutter M, Le Couteur A. Autism diagnostic interview-revised: a revised version of a diagnostic interview for caregivers of individuals with possible pervasive developmental disorders. J Autism Dev Disord 1994;24(5):659–85.
53. Greenspan SI, Serena W. A functional developmental approach to autism spectrum disorders. Res Pract Persons Severe Disabl 1999;24(3):147–61.

Early Identification and Treatment of Antisocial Behavior

Paul J. Frick, PhD[a,b,*]

KEYWORDS

- Antisocial behavior • Early identification • Treatment • Callous-unemotional traits
- Emotional regulation • Diagnosis

KEY POINTS

- Individuals most likely to show severe and persistent antisocial behavior often begin showing severe conduct problems early in childhood.
- Callous-unemotional (CU) traits are characterized by a lack of guilt, a lack of empathy, a restricted display of affect, and a failure to put forth the effort to succeed in important activities.
- The level of CU traits seems to differentiate subgroups of children and adolescents with serious conduct problems who differ in the severity and persistence of their antisocial behavior.
- The level of CU traits also seems to differentiate subgroups of children and adolescents with serious conduct who have different causes to their behavior problems.
- Treatment is enhanced when it is tailored to the unique characteristics of antisocial youth with and without elevated CU traits.

INTRODUCTION

Antisocial behavior in children and adolescents is generally defined by behavior that violates the rights of others, such as aggression, destruction of property, and theft; or behavior that violates major age-appropriate societal norms or rules, such as truancy and running away from home.[1] Serious and persistent patterns of antisocial behavior in children and adolescents form the diagnostic criteria for conduct disorder (CD),[1] and CD is a critical mental health concern for several reasons:

- It is highly prevalent with a worldwide prevalence among children and adolescents ages 6 to 18 estimated at 3.2%.[2]

Disclosure Statement: The author has nothing to disclose.
[a] Department of Psychology, Louisiana State University, Baton Rouge, LA 70802, USA; [b] Learning Sciences Institute of Australia, Australian Catholic University, Melbourne, VIC, Australia
* Department of Psychology, Louisiana State University, Baton Rouge, LA 70802.
E-mail address: pfrick@lsu.edu

- It operates at a high cost to society because of the reduced quality of life for the victims of the antisocial acts and the financial costs to the legal system that must respond to the acts that violate laws.[3]
- It predicts a host of problems in adjustment for the person with the disorder throughout their lifespan, including mental health problems (eg, substance abuse), legal problems (eg, risk for arrest), educational problems (eg, school dropout), social problems (eg, poor marital adjustment), occupational problems (eg, poor job performance), and physical health problems (eg, poor respiratory function).[4]

Given the prevalence, cost, and impairment associated with CD, it is not surprising that a substantial amount of research has been conducted to understand the causes of this disorder and to use this knowledge to develop effective methods to prevent or treat it. One of the most consistent findings from this work is that interventions that seek to target a reduction in antisocial behavior are least costly and most effective if they are implemented early in childhood.[5] As a result, a substantial amount of research on CD has focused on identifying early markers that predict either who will develop the disorder or who is at risk for showing the most severe and persistent forms of antisocial behavior once it develops.

BEHAVIORAL APPROACHES TO EARLY IDENTIFICATION
Types of Behavior Associated with Poor Outcomes

Early research attempting to identify early indicators of risk for persistent antisocial behavior focused on the frequency and severity of the behavior displayed, with severity being defined as the number and variety of different behaviors displayed by the child and the number of settings in which the child displays the behaviors.[6] For example, Robins reported on a classic longitudinal study of 314 children referred to a child mental health clinic for CD symptoms and reported that the risk for showing an antisocial disorder as an adult was a linear function of the number of symptoms exhibited in childhood.[7] Specifically, 15% of children with 3 to 5 symptoms in childhood were diagnosed with an antisocial disorder as an adult, in comparison to 25% of children with 6 or 7 symptoms, 29% of children with 8 or 9 symptoms, and 43% of children with greater than 10 symptoms.

Another early marker of severity for children and adolescents with CD has been the presence of aggression. That is, when antisocial behavior is separated into those behaviors that can be considered aggressive (eg, bullies others, initiates physical fights) and those that are nonaggressive (eg, vandalism, lies, truant), the aggressive behaviors seem to be more stable and stronger predictors of problems continuing into adulthood.[8] In addition to simply documenting the presence of aggression, there has been research suggesting that the form that the aggression takes could be important. For example, research has distinguished between reactive aggression, which occurs as an angry response to provocation or threat, and proactive aggression, which is typically unprovoked and often used for instrumental gain or dominance over others.[9] Research suggests that some children with severe conduct problems only show reactive forms of aggression, whereas others show a combination of both reactive and proactive forms of aggression.[10] Children showing combined forms of aggression often have more problems across development.[9]

Thus, research suggests that the number, severity, and degree of harm that a child's antisocial behavior causes to others are important factors to consider as markers of risk for poor outcome. To reflect this, the diagnostic criteria for CD in the most recent editions of the Diagnostic and Statistical Manual of Mental Disorders (DSM)[1,11] have required that the person must show at least 3 different antisocial behaviors over the past 12 months to be diagnosed with CD, and then the severity is coded as:

- *Mild:* with few symptoms beyond the diagnostic threshold and behavior that causes relative minor harm to others (eg, lying, truancy);
- *Moderate:* the number of symptoms and amount of harm to others is intermediate to those specified as "mild" or "severe";
- *Severe:* many symptoms beyond the diagnostic threshold that cause considerable harm to others (eg, rape, use of a weapon).

Childhood Onset Conduct Disorder

Another important variation in how antisocial behavior is expressed in children is the age at which the serious antisocial behavior is first displayed. Persons who begin showing behavior problems before adolescence are much more likely to continue to show problems into adulthood compared with those whose problems onset during adolescence. For example, in a birth cohort from New Zealand that was followed into adulthood, the rate of official convictions for violent acts in adulthood (before age 32) was as follows:

- 32.7% for males who began showing serious conduct problems before adolescence
- 10.2% for males who began showing serious conduct problems in adolescence
- .4% for males who did not show serious conduct problems in either childhood or adolescence.[4]

Even before adolescence, there is some indication that the younger the child begins to show serious conduct problems, the more severe and persistent his or her antisocial behavior is likely to be.[12] Importantly, the age of onset of antisocial behavior may subsume some of the other behavioral patterns that predict poor outcomes. That is, age of onset is negatively associated with number of conduct problems and with the level of aggression displayed by the child.[12,13]

As a result of this research, the most recent editions of the DSM have also included criteria to distinguish early and late onset patterns of CD:

- *Childhood-onset type*: Individuals show at least one symptom characteristic of CD before age 10 years.
- *Adolescent-onset type*: Individuals show no symptom characteristic of CD before age 10 years.[1]

The different outcomes for these 2 subgroups of antisocial individuals may be due to differences in the causal processes that lead to the different trajectories.[13,14] Specifically, the childhood-onset pattern seems to be more strongly related to neuropsychological (eg, deficits in executive functioning) and cognitive (eg, low intelligence) deficits. Also, children who show the childhood-onset pattern seem to show more temperamental and personality risk factors, such as impulsivity, attention deficits, and problems in emotional regulation. As a result, this group often displays attention-deficit hyperactivity disorder (ADHD), and it is possible that the presence of ADHD contributes to their poor outcomes.[15] Importantly for early identification, the impulsivity and hyperactivity symptoms of ADHD often emerge before the child's conduct problems and can be the first indicator that the child is having problems regulating their behavior and emotions.[15]

In contrast to this early-onset trajectory, persons whose antisocial behavior onsets in adolescence typically do not show the same number and severity of dispositional risk factors, like ADHD.[13,14] However, they are often described as showing higher levels of rebelliousness and being more rejecting of conventional values and status hierarchies.[16] As a result, youths in the adolescent-onset pathway are often considered as showing an exaggeration of the normative process of adolescent rebellion in which the adolescent engages in antisocial and delinquent behaviors as a misguided attempt to obtain a subjective sense of maturity and adult status in a way that is maladaptive (eg, breaking societal norms) but encouraged by an antisocial peer group.[4]

CALLOUS-UNEMOTIONAL TRAITS AND DEVELOPMENTAL PATHWAYS TO ANTISOCIAL BEHAVIOR

All of these approaches to identifying children who are at most risk for showing persistent antisocial behavior have focused on some aspect of how the antisocial behavior is expressed (ie, number, type, or onset of the behavior). However, there is another approach that focuses instead on the person's affective and interpersonal style, similar to definitions of psychopathy in adults.[17] This style has been labeled as "callous-unemotional (CU) traits" in research[18] and as "limited prosocial emotions" in diagnostic criteria for CD.[1] Specifically, the 5th edition of the DSM includes a specifier (ie, "With Limited Prosocial Emotions") that can be applied to persons who meet criteria for CD but who show at least 2 of the following symptoms over an extended period of time (ie, at least 12 months) and in multiple relationships and settings:

- Lack for remorse or guilt
- Callous-lack of empathy
- Unconcerned about performance in important activities
- Shallow or deficient affect.

These specific indicators and the diagnostic threshold of 2 symptoms were chosen based on extensive secondary data analyses across large samples of youth in different countries.[19] Importantly, although only a minority (25%–30%) of children with CD meets the criteria for this specifier, this group seems to differ from other antisocial youth in many important ways.[18]

Differences Between Conduct Disorder with and Without Elevated Callous-UnemotionalTraits

In terms of clinical importance, antisocial youth with CU traits (relative to other antisocial youth) show the following:

- A more stable pattern of antisocial behavior that predicts a greater likelihood of the antisocial behavior continuing into adulthood[20,21]
- More severe aggression that results in greater harm to others[22,23]
- Aggression that is more likely to be premeditated and instrumental (ie, for personal gain and dominance)[22–24]
- Poorer response to many of the typical health interventions used to treat CD.[25,26]

Thus, the presence of elevated CU traits identifies a group of antisocial youth who are important for early intervention and treatment.

In addition, there is evidence that these traits also classify a group of youth with CD who show very different genetic, cognitive, emotional, and social characteristics from other antisocial youth.[18] Specifically, antisocial youth with elevated CU traits (relative to other antisocial children and adolescents):

- Show stronger genetic influences on their conduct problem behavior[27]
- Show an insensitivity to punishment cues under many conditions[28]

- View aggression as a more acceptable means for obtaining goals and place greater importance on dominance and revenge in social conflicts[29]
- Display reduced emotional responses to cues of distress in others[30,31]
- Show impairments in their selective attention to caregivers face in the first year of life, make less eye contact with caregivers in childhood, and attend less to the eye region in others later in life[32–34]
- Show conduct problems that are less related to hostile and coercive parenting but are more strongly related to warm parenting[35]
- Are more likely to associate with deviant peers, are more likely to commit crimes with peers, and are more influential in encouraging antisocial behavior in their peers.[36,37]

This extensive list of differences between antisocial youth with and without elevated CU traits has led to several theories proposing different causes to the antisocial behavior in the 2 groups. For example, children with serious conduct problems and elevated CU traits have a temperament that could make them more difficult to socialize (eg, less sensitive punishment) and miss early signs of distress in others (eg, reduced emotional responses to others' distress).[38] These processes can interfere with the normal development of key aspects of conscience (ie, empathy and guilt) and place the child at risk for a particularly severe and aggressive pattern of antisocial behavior.

In contrast, children with childhood-onset antisocial behavior with normative levels

- Are highly reactive to emotional cues in others
- Are highly distressed by the effects of their behavior on others
- Display higher levels of emotional reactivity to provocation from others.

They show conduct problems that are

- Less strongly influenced by genetic factors
- More strongly associated with hostile/coercive parenting.[14,18]

Based on these findings, It appears that children in this group show a temperament characterized by strong emotional reactivity combined with inadequate socializing experiences that lead to failure in the development of the skills needed to adequately regulate their emotional reactivity.[39,40] The resulting problems in emotional regulation can result in the child committing impulsive and unplanned aggressive and antisocial acts, for which he or she may feel remorseful afterward, but for which he or she may still have difficulty controlling in the future.

Implications for Research

From this brief review of research, it is clear that the distinction between antisocial youth with and without elevated CU traits may encompass several of the previous attempts to define important subgroups of children at risk for particularly severe and stable patterns of antisocial behavior. Specifically, children with elevated CU traits and conduct problems tend to show a greater number of conduct problems, more aggressive behavior, and more instrumental aggression.[18] Furthermore, CU traits seem to designate a subgroup of children within those with both ADHD and early conduct problems who show distinct emotional and cognitive characteristics[41] and who are at particularly high risk for later antisocial behavior.[21] With respect to the latter, McMahon and colleagues[21] reported that CU traits assessed in seventh grade significantly predicted adult antisocial outcomes (eg, adult arrests, adult antisocial personality symptoms) even after controlling for ADHD, oppositional defiant disorder, CD, and childhood-onset of CD.

The presence of elevated CU traits seems particularly important for guiding research investigating the causes of antisocial behavior because they differentiate groups with very different emotional and cognitive characteristics. To illustrate this, Viding and colleagues[31] reported that amygdala responses to fearful faces (relative to calm faces) were stronger in boys (ages 10–16) with conduct problems without elevated CU traits but were weaker in boys with conduct problems who were elevated on CU traits compared with controls. Thus, ignoring the differences among the 2 groups high on conduct problems would have hidden the differences with controls and led to erroneous conclusions on the potential importance of emotional responding for understanding the development of conduct problems.

Another way that research on CU traits could be critical for causal theories of antisocial behavior is that it promotes an integration of research on processes in typically developing children with research on how these developmental processes can go awry and lead to problem behavior.[38] As noted above, many theories to explain the differences between antisocial youth with and without elevated CU traits include processes that have long been the focus of developmental research, such as how children develop guilt, empathy, and other prosocial emotions and how children develop the skills necessary to regulate their emotions.[40] Thus, causal theories for antisocial behavior can be advanced by integrating it with the vast research on conscience development and the development of emotional regulation in non-antisocial children.

Furthermore, this approach to research on antisocial behavior in children and adolescents would be consistent with the research domain criteria (R-DoC) framework that is being advanced by the National Institute of Mental Health. Specifically, the R-DoC initiative was implemented to overcome some of the limitations in behaviorally based approaches to classifying mental health disorders, such as the great heterogeneity in the neurocognitive mechanisms that can lead to a single behavioral diagnosis like CD.[42] As noted above, the use of CU traits seems to reduce this heterogeneity by designating groups with similar behavioral manifestations (ie, CD) but with unique profiles of neurocognitive processes.[39] Furthermore, these neurocognitive profiles can be explained using the R-DoC domains, with the group without elevated CU traits showing problems in the regulation of the negative emotional valence system responsible for responses to aversive situations and contexts (eg, anxiety, frustration, and loss) and the group with elevated CU traits showing problems primarily in the systems for social processing that mediate responses to interpersonal settings, especially related to affiliation and attachment.[42] Thus, advances in knowledge of the RDoC domains could be critical for guiding research on how these domains may be related to the development of antisocial behavior.

Implications for Prevention and Treatment

The research on CU traits and the different developmental pathways to antisocial behavior could also have many important implications for preventing and treating CD. Existing research on effective treatments for antisocial behavior in children and adolescents highlights the need to

- Intervene as early in development as possible
- Intervene with comprehensive treatments that target many dispositional and contextual risk factors that can lead to or maintain the child's antisocial behavior
- Tailor interventions to the unique needs of children and adolescents with serious antisocial behavior, because the most important targets of intervention may vary across antisocial individuals.[43]

Research on the differences between antisocial children and adolescents with and without elevated CU traits can advance each of these goals.

For example, as noted above, the most effective treatments for antisocial behavior intervene early in development when the child's conduct problems are less severe.[43] The research on the different developmental mechanisms leading to CD could allow interventions to target children who show temperamental vulnerabilities (eg, children who miss early cues to others' distress or who have problems regulating their emotions) even before the serious conduct problems develop.[44,45] Furthermore, parenting interventions could be modified to meet the unique needs of these children with very different temperaments.[46]

This ability to tailor treatments to the needs of the different youth with CD could be the most important benefit of recognizing the various developmental pathways to antisocial behavior. That is, the different characteristics associated with antisocial behavior in those with and without elevated CU traits could help in determining the most effective combination of services for an individual child or adolescent. As noted previously, children and adolescents who show significant levels of CU traits present quite a treatment challenge.[18] However, despite their poor response to many traditional treatments, their antisocial behavior can be reduced when intensive treatments are tailored to their unique cognitive and emotional characteristics.

For example, Hawes and Dadds[26] reported that clinic-referred boys (ages 4–9) with conduct problems and elevated CU traits showed reductions in their conduct problems during the phase of a parenting intervention that focused on use of positive reinforcement to encourage prosocial behavior. This outcome would be consistent with the reward-oriented response style that appears to be characteristic of children with CU traits. Similarly, Caldwell and colleagues[47] demonstrated that adolescent offenders with CU traits improved (ie, showed significant reductions in reoffending) when treated using an intensive treatment program that used reward-oriented approaches, targeted the self-interests of the adolescent, and taught empathy skills. Finally, White and colleagues[48] tested the effectiveness of an intervention for adolescents in the juvenile justice system that focused on engaging the child and family in treatment and providing motivations for change that are individualized for each family and child. Results indicated that CU traits were associated with improvements in behavior over the course of treatment and with decreases in risk for reoffending at 6- and 12-month follow-ups. Thus, certain treatments can reduce the level and severity of the antisocial behavior of youths with CU traits, if they are tailored to the unique characteristics of this group.

SUMMARY

In summary, severe and persistent antisocial behavior is a serious and costly mental health problem. Persistently antisocial individuals often start showing conduct problems early in development, and interventions that seek to treat these problems before they worsen are the most effective and least costly. Thus, early intervention for serious conduct problems is a critical goal for reducing the burden of antisocial behavior on individuals and society. Furthermore, research has suggested that there are likely several important causal pathways that lead to severe and persistent antisocial behavior. One pathway involves a failure to develop appropriate levels of empathy, guilt, and other aspects of conscience that leads to severe aggression that is planned and instrumental in nature. Another pathway involves a failure to develop adequate emotional regulation that leads to impulsive aggressive acts or other antisocial behaviors during periods of intense emotional arousal that interfere with the child's ability to adequately consider the consequences of his or her behavior. These developmental pathways respond differently to treatment, and the most effective treatments are tailored to the unique characteristics of individuals in the various groups.

This framework for understanding serious conduct problems in youths is important for guiding research by illustrating the need to use designs and statistical procedures that can capture the different associations with important causal variables across the different pathways. Furthermore, the unique pattern of neurocognitive processes underlying these different pathways fits well with the RDoC framework. As suggested by this framework, prospective studies in which children are grouped according to the different patterns of emotional, cognitive, and biological variables and then are followed to track the onset of conduct problems could be critical for advancing causal theory. Within such a research design, testing potential contextual factors that could moderate the risk for antisocial behavior in youth with certain types of neurocognitive risk could be critical for advancing interventions. For example, research suggests that warm and responsive parenting may reduce the level of CU traits in children who are temperamentally vulnerable to missing signs of distress in others.[49] Such findings can be used to enhance existing treatments and lead to better outcomes for children and adolescents who heretofore have been resistant to typical mental health treatments. Finally, now that these pathways have been integrated into diagnostic criteria, it is likely that these distinctions among subgroups of youth with CD will be made more commonly in clinical settings, and research is needed to develop and test valid and cost-efficient means for making these distinctions.[50]

REFERENCES

1. American Psychiatric Association. Diagnostic and statistical manual of mental disorders. 5th edition. Washington, DC: American Psychiatric Association; 2013.
2. Canino G, Polanczyk G, Bauermeister JJ, et al. Does the prevalence of CD and ODD vary across cultures? Soc Psychiatry Psychiatr Epidemiol 2010;45:695–704.
3. Cohen MA, Piquero AR. New evidence on the monetary value of saving a high risk youth. J Quant Criminol 2009;25:25–49.
4. Odgers DL, Caspi A, Broadbent JM, et al. Prediction of differential adult health burden by conduct problem subtypes in males. Arch Gen Psychiatry 2007;64: 476–84.
5. Eyberg SM, Nelson MM, Boggs SR. Evidence-based psychosocial treatments for children and adolescents with disruptive behavior. J Clin Child Adolesc Psychol 2008;37:215–37.
6. Loeber R. Antisocial behavior: more enduring than changeable? J Am Acad Child Adolesc Psychiatry 1991;30:393–7.
7. Robins LN. Deviant children grown up. Baltimore (MD): Williams and Wilkins; 1966.
8. Hyde LW, Burt SA, Shaw DS, et al. Early starting, aggressive, and/or callous-unemotional? Examining the overlap and predictive utility of antisocial behavior subtypes. J Abnorm Psychol 2015;124:329–42.
9. Marsee MA, Frick PJ. Callous-unemotional traits and aggression in youth. In: Arsenio WF, Lemerise EA, editors. Emotions, aggression and morality in children. Washington, DC: American Psychological Association; 2010. p. 137–56.
10. Marsee MA, Frick PJ, Barry CT, et al. Profiles of forms and functions of self-reported aggression in three adolescent samples. Dev Psychopathol 2014;26: 705–20.
11. American Psychiatric Association. Diagnostic and statistical manual of mental disorders. 4th edition. Washington, DC: American Psychiatric Association; 1994.

12. Lahey BB, Goodman SH, Waldman ID, et al. Relation of age of onset to the type and severity of child and adolescent conduct problems. J Abnorm Child Psychol 1999;27:247–60.

13. Moffitt TE. Life-course persistent versus adolescence-limited antisocial behavior. In: Cicchetti D, Cohen DJ, editors. Developmental psychopathology, 2nd edition, vol. 3: risk, disorder, and adaptation. New York: Wiley; 2006. p. 570–98.

14. Frick PJ, Viding EM. Antisocial behavior from a developmental psychopathology perspective. Dev Psychopathol 2009;21:1111–31.

15. Waschbusch DA. A meta-analytic examination of comorbid hyperactive-impulsive-attention problems and conduct problems. Psychol Bull 2002;128:118–50.

16. Dandreaux DM, Frick PJ. Developmental pathways to conduct problems: a further test of the childhood and adolescent-onset distinction. J Abnorm Child Psychol 2009;37:375–85.

17. Hare RD, Neumann CS. Psychopath as a clinical and empirical construct. Annu Rev Clin Psychol 2008;4:217–46.

18. Frick PJ, Ray JV, Thornton LC, et al. Can callous-unemotional traits enhance the understanding, diagnosis, and treatment of serious conduct problems in children and adolescents? A comprehensive review. Psychol Bull 2014;140:1–57.

19. Kimonis ER, Fanti KA, Frick PJ, et al. Using self-reported callous-unemotional traits to cross-nationally assess the DSM-5 "With Limited Prosocial Emotions" specifier. J Child Psychol Psychiatry 2015;56:1249–61.

20. Frick PJ, Stickle TR, Dandreaux DM, et al. Callous-unemotional traits in predicting the severity and stability of conduct problems and delinquency. J Abnorm Child Psychol 2005;33:471–87.

21. McMahon RJ, Witkiewitz K, Kotler JS, Conduct Problems Prevention Research Group. Predictive validity of callous-unemotional traits measures in early adolescence with respect to multiple antisocial outcomes. J Abnorm Psychol 2010;119:752–63.

22. Kruh IP, Frick PJ, Clements CB. Historical and personality correlates to the violence patterns of juveniles tried as adults. Crim Justice Behav 2005;32:69–96.

23. Lawing K, Frick PJ, Cruise KR. Differences in offending patterns between adolescent sex offenders high or low in callous-unemotional traits. Psychol Assess 2010;22:298–305.

24. Frick PJ, Cornell AH, Barry CT, et al. Callous-unemotional traits and conduct problems in the prediction of conduct problem severity, aggression, and self-report of delinquency. J Abnorm Child Psychol 2003;31:457–70.

25. Haas SM, Waschbusch DA, Pelham WE, et al. Treatment response in CP/ADHD children with callous/unemotional traits. J Abnorm Child Psychol 2011;4:541–52.

26. Hawes DJ, Dadds MR. he treatment of conduct problems in children with callous-unemotional traits. J Consult Clin Psychol 2005;73:737–41.

27. Viding E, Jones AP, Frick PJ, et al. Heritability of antisocial behaviour at 9: do callous-unemotional traits matter? Dev Sci 2008;11:17–22.

28. Blair RJ, Colledge E, Murray L, et al. A selective impairment in the processing of sad and fearful expressions in children with psychopathic tendencies. J Abnorm Child Psychol 2001;29:491–8.

29. Pardini DA, Lochman JE, Frick PJ. Callous-unemotional traits and social-cognitive processes in adjudicated youths. J Am Acad Child Adolesc Psychiatry 2003;42:364–71.

30. Kimonis ER, Frick PJ, Fazekas H, et al. Psychopathy, aggression, and the emotional processing of emotional stimuli in non-referred girls and boys. Behav Sci Law 2006;24:21–37.

31. Viding E, Sebastian CL, Dadds MR, et al. Amygdala response to preattentive masked fear in children with conduct problems: the role of callous-unemotional traits. Am J Psychiatry 2012;169:1109–16.

32. Bedford R, Pickles A, Sharp H, et al. Reduced face preference in infancy: a developmental precursor to callous-unemotional traits? Biol Psychiatry 2015;78:144–50.

33. Dadds MR, El Masry Y, Wimalaweera S, et al. Reduced eye gaze explains "fear blindness" in childhood psychopathic traits. J Am Acad Child Adolesc Psychiatry 2008;47:455–63.

34. Dadds MR, Jabrak J, Pasalich D, et al. Impaired attention to the eyes of attachment figures and the developmental origins of psychopathy. J Child Psychol Psychiatry 2011;52:238–45.

35. Pasalich DS, Dadds MR, Hawes DJ, et al. Do callous-unemotional traits moderate the relative importance of parental coercion versus warmth in child conduct problems? An observational study. J Child Psychol Psychiatry 2012;52:1308–15.

36. Kerr M, Van Zalk M, Stattin H. Psychopathic traits moderate peer influence on adolescent delinquency. J Child Psychol Psychiatry 2012;53:826–35.

37. Thornton LC, Frick PJ, Shulman EP, et al. Callous-unemotional traits and adolescents' role in group crime. Law Hum Behav 2015;39:368–77.

38. Frick PJ, Ray JV, Thornton LC, et al. Annual research review: a developmental psychopathology approach to understanding callous-unemotional traits in children and adolescents with serious conduct problems. J Child Psychol Psychiatry 2014;55:532–48.

39. Blair RJR. Empathy, moral development, and aggression: a cognitive neuroscience perspective. In: Arsenio WF, Lemerise EA, editors. Emotions, aggression and morality in children. Washington, DC: American Psychological Association; 2010. p. 97–114.

40. Frick PJ, Morris AS. Temperament and developmental pathways to conduct problems. J Clin Child Adolesc Psychol 2004;33:54–68.

41. Barry CT, Frick PJ, Grooms T, et al. The importance of callous-unemotional traits for extending the concept of psychopathy to children. J Abnorm Psychol 2000;109:335–40.

42. Insel T, Cuthbert B, Garvey M, et al. Research domain criteria (RDoC): toward a new classification framework for research on mental disorders. Am J Psychiatry 2010;167:748–51.

43. Frick PJ. Developmental pathways to conduct disorder: implication for future directions in research, assessment, and treatment. J Clin Child Adolesc Psychol 2012;42:378–89.

44. Dadds MR, Allen JL, McGregor K, et al. Callous-unemotional traits in children and mechanisms of impaired eye contact during expressions of love: a treatment target? J Child Psychol Psychiatry 2014;55:771–80.

45. Kochanska G, Kim S, Boldt LJ, et al. Promoting toddlers' positive social-emotional outcomes in low-income families: a play-based experimental study. J Clin Child Adolesc Psychol 2013;42:700–12.

46. Kimonis ER, Armstrong K. Adapting parent-child interaction therapy to treat severe conduct problems with callous-unemotional traits: a case study. Clin Case Stud 2012;11:234–52.

47. Caldwell M, Skeem J, Salekin R, et al. Treatment response of adolescent offenders with psychopathy features: a 2-year follow-up. Crim Justice Behav 2006;33:571–96.

48. White SF, Frick PJ, Lawing SK, et al. Callous-unemotional traits and response to functional family therapy in adolescent offenders. Behav Sci Law 2013;31: 271–85.
49. Waller R, Gardner F, Hyde LW. What are the associations between parenting, callous-unemotional traits, and antisocial behavior in youth? A systematic review of evidence. Clin Psychol Rev 2013;33:593–608.
50. Frick PJ, Ray JV. Evaluating callous-unemotional traits as a personality construct. J Pers 2015;83:710–22.

Specialized Behavioral Therapies for Children with Special Needs

Susan G. Timmer, PhD*, Anthony J. Urquiza, PhD

KEYWORDS

- Child trauma • Evidence-based treatments • Maltreated children & adolescents
- Therapeutic interventions • Child development

KEY POINTS

- The quality of a child's environment, along with age and developmental stage, can shape mental health outcomes and the way the child views the world.
- Chronic stress in children and the experience of adverse childhood events can affect brain development, stress hormone production, and other physiologic systems.
- Positive and responsive caregiving is important for emotion regulation and mental health in infants and toddlers.
- Interventions for middle childhood and adolescence focus on the child's perceptions and emotions and aim to increase safety through positive social and family support.

INTRODUCTION

In their "Mental Health Surveillance Among Children, 2005–2011," the Centers for Disease Control and Prevention (CDC)[1] reported that between 13% and 20% of children in the United States experience a mental health disorder in a year. Other data from the CDC suggest that only about a third of children whose parents spoke to a health care provider or school staff about their emotional or behavioral difficulties will receive specialized behavioral treatment for these concerns.[2] One cannot help but wonder why so many children go untreated. Is it because the problems mentioned are not recognized as warranting intervention? Is it because health care providers and school staff do not know what kinds of services in their communities might help these families?

The purpose of this article is to describe common mental health problems in children and adolescents, and the types of specialized, evidence-based behavioral

CAARE Diagnostic and Treatment Center, UC Davis Children's Hospital, Department of Pediatrics, 3671 Business Drive, Sacramento, CA 95820, USA
* Corresponding author. Department of Pediatrics, CAARE Diagnostic & Treatment Center, UC Davis Children's Hospital, 3671 Business Drive, Sacramento, CA 95820.
E-mail address: stimmer@ucdavis.edu

Pediatr Clin N Am 63 (2016) 873–885
http://dx.doi.org/10.1016/j.pcl.2016.06.012   pediatric.theclinics.com
0031-3955/16/$ – see front matter © 2016 Elsevier Inc. All rights reserved.

treatments that are most effective in treating these needs. These descriptions are followed by illustrations of a select number of well-researched interventions that address many of these problems.

What Causes Mental Health Problems in Children?

There is no single cause of mental health problems in children. Theory about how mental health problems develop proposes that different qualities of children's environments—their cultural environments, social resources, family environments, and individual differences—shape the way children respond to the surrounding world.[3] The characteristics of their environments influence children's ability to grow and mature, providing emotional support and cognitive frameworks at one point in time, which influence later development. The child's environment is seen as having "potentiating factors" that increase the child's vulnerability, and "compensatory factors" that increase resilience.

So far, this model seems simple—the ratio of positives to negatives in the child's environment predicts the likelihood of mental health problems. However, a negative event occurring when the child is 2 years old can have a different effect on the child's mental health from the same event occurring when the child is 5 years old. Two and 5 year olds differ considerably in cognitive ability, which might affect the following:

- Their likelihood of noticing a traumatic event
- The meaning they would attach to the event
- The degree to which the event's meaning would be linked to the child's perception of self, emotional security, or physical safety
- Their ability to verbalize distress
- The effect of their distress on behavior

Maturation is thought to drive reorganization of previous experiences, prompting children to adopt a more complex understanding of their environment and life history. However, even in the face of adverse events, environmental stress, or neurobiological predisposition, it is always possible for children to build resilience and improve functioning. What this means is that changing the trajectory of development is possible when there is new experience, particularly when new, positive experiences force reorganization of old negative experiences and thought patterns. It also means that effective mental health interventions can help modify the negative effects of early adversity.

Traumatic Events and the Developing Child

One tends to think that infants are safe from the most devastating effects of traumatic events or circumstances. We do not remember our first several years, so we might assume that infants will not remember adverse events. Nevertheless, accumulating evidence suggests that chronic exposure to fear and anxiety and abusive caregiving leaves a neurologic footprint.[4]

Chronic or acute stress, possibly resulting from maltreatment or other adverse childhood experiences (ACEs), described in **Fig. 1**, can activate or inhibit other physiologic systems involved in the stress response. When infants are chronically exposed to stress hormones, the body's feedback systems for managing and regulating stress hormone production can become dysregulated, which increases their physiologic vulnerability.[5] This increased vulnerability may create challenges with emotional, cognitive, and physical health.[6] The take-away message of this research, illustrated in **Fig. 2**, is that early trauma affects the way children will respond to future stressful

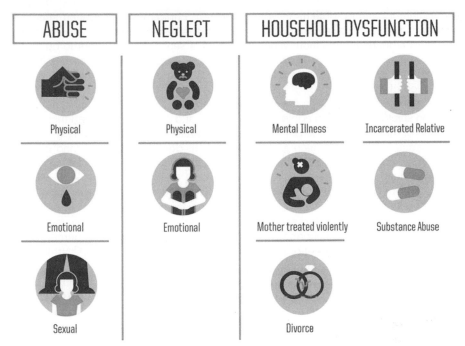

Fig. 1. The 3 types of ACEs. (*Courtesy of* Robert Wood Johnson Foundation, Princeton, NJ. Copyright 2015; with permission.)

events. Furthermore, the way they respond makes them vulnerable to difficulties and delays that create other problems later in development.

In addition to the clear effects of trauma and maltreatment on children, parents' interpersonal and parenting styles also affect children's health and mental health. Parents' mental health problems have been found to disrupt healthy development.[4] Children of depressed mothers are reported to have more behavior problems[7] and a higher risk of later psychopathology.[8]

Taken all together, research suggests that in the early years, emotional dysregulation resulting from attempts to manage the anxiety of perceived threats is at the root of

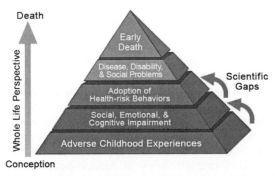

Fig. 2. The ACEs pyramid. (*Courtesy of* Robert Wood Johnson Foundation, Princeton, NJ. Copyright 2015; with permission.)

many mental health problems in young children. Furthermore, parenting seems to directly influence the stress response system and is key to children's developing capacity for emotional regulation. When parenting is sensitive, it appears to buffer the effects of stress on children.[9] When parenting is ineffective and nonoptimal, it magnifies the stressfulness of early traumatic experiences, possibly by increasing the perception of threat.[10]

One of the most widely documented effects of ACEs is an increased risk of depression and suicidal ideation in adolescence.[11] Dube and colleagues[11] found that among a cohort of more than 17,000 primary care clinic patients, having a history of adverse experiences in childhood such as abuse, neglect, domestic violence, and parents' substance abuse doubled to quintupled the likelihood of attempted suicide in adolescence.

Apart from the physical growth and cognitive maturity that takes place from childhood to adolescence, the way children interpret events in the world around them changes dramatically. An increasing number of studies connect early adverse experiences with differences in cognitions and perceptions, including the perception of emotion in others,[12] perceptions of the causes of emotional states,[13] attributions about traumatic events,[14] attention to social information and peer behavior,[15] and perceptions of their control over events.[16] These findings combine to suggest that cognition and meaning play significant roles in adolescent mental health, in a way that it does not in younger children.

INTERVENTIONS FOR INFANTS

Infant mental health is based on factors that promote biological and emotional regulation, and emotional security in infants and toddlers. Neurologic and biological child characteristics play a part in determining their mental health. However, parents' responses to infants' behavior and parents' own mental health also moderate these symptoms. Likely for this reason, almost all interventions for infants focus primarily on parents' behaviors and attachment mindedness. Attachment and biobehavioral catch-up[17] (ABC) is one such intervention with a strong evidence base. Multiple randomized controlled trials (RCTs) support the efficacy of ABC in improving CPS-referred infants' and toddlers' attachment to their caregivers and physiologic stress.[9]

Attachment and Biobehavioral Catch-Up

Guiding principles
This intervention focuses on improving parents' responsiveness and the predictability of infant and toddlers' caregiving environment, thereby improving children's attachment quality, emotional, behavioral, and biobehavioral regulation.

Goals of treatment
Three primary goals or components are identified. In component A, caregivers (adoptive, foster, or biological) learn the meaning of infants' rejecting cues. The caregivers practice nurturing skills even when the children fail to ask for comfort or reject their attempts to provide comfort. In component B, caregivers learn new strategies for reacting to children's distress. Adapted from child parent psychotherapy,[18] therapists intervene to help caregivers recognize their own attachment-related issues that interfere with their ability to nurture their children and help them to become more responsive. In component C, therapists work to reduce behavioral and biobehavioral dysregulation by creating a caregiving environment that is predictable, responsive, and child-centered.

Strategies for achieving goals
The intervention is designed for the parents of children between 10 and 24 months of age, but can be modified for different aged children. Treatment is conducted over 10 sessions, each lasting about an hour, in the family's home. Therapists use a daily diary to find out about the child's behavior, and the parent's and child's contingent behavior; they use video to record the parent and child interacting for supervisorial review and to show the caregiver their progress in treatment.

Caregivers first learn the basic concepts of the intervention and then collaboratively analyze and reframe the child's attachment cues. In the subsequent 2 sessions, therapists explore attachment issues that may interfere with the parent's ability to respond positively to the infant. Once the attachment-related reactions have been discussed, therapists discuss and practice the importance of positive physical touch for the infant. In the ninth session, therapists teach caregivers to read and respond effectively to children's emotional cues. They review information and wrap up in the tenth session.

INTERVENTIONS FOR YOUNG CHILDREN

As in infancy, parents play a key role in determining their young children's mental health. Intensive interventions for young children typically involve parents, teaching parents positive parenting skills either while playing with their children one on one or in a parent-group setting. These interventions use different methods of delivery but their purposes are similar: to teach parents skills to improve the parenting environment for the child and to help them better manage their children's difficult behaviors. They are primarily designed for young children in approximately the 2- to 8-year age range and their parents, but often are provided to somewhat older children.

There are many excellent interventions for young children. Eighteen interventions are listed in Substance Abuse and Mental Health Services Administration's *Evidence Based Practice Kit*[19]; among them is the Parent-Child Interaction Therapy (PCIT).[20] PCIT is one of the few interventions that uses an individual therapy modality and fully involves both the parent and the child in therapy sessions.

Parent-Child Interaction Therapy

Guiding principles
Like many parenting-oriented interventions, PCIT is founded on the belief that the parent's attention must be a source of reward for the child before behavior management strategies can be effective. PCIT works toward increasing parents' attention to their children's positive behaviors for this reason. At the same time, PCIT emphasizes the power of changing behavioral mechanics as a way to improve the emotional quality of the interaction.

Goals of treatment
Although the child is the *client* in treatment, and reducing disruptive behaviors is the *goal* of PCIT, parents' behaviors are the real target. Therapists coach parents to be more positive and consistent and to use predictable behavior management strategies. When they accomplish these goals, they become the agent of change in reducing their child's behavior problems.

Strategies for achieving goals
PCIT incorporates both parent and child (aged 2–7 years old) in the treatment sessions and uses live therapist "coaching" for an individualized approach to adjusting the malfunctioning parent-child relationship. Treatment is conducted in 2 phases over 14 to

20 weeks. Both phases of treatment begin with an hour of didactic training, when parents are taught and practice specific skills of communication and behavior management with their children. Teaching sessions are followed by sessions in which the therapist coaches the parent during play with the child. In the clinic, therapists coach from an observation room behind a 2-way mirror via a frequency modulation receiver, providing the parent with feedback on their use of skills, as shown in **Fig. 3**.

In the first phase (child-directed interaction; CDI), the therapist works to enhance the parent-child relationship. By the end of CDI, parents generally have shifted from rarely noticing their children's positive behavior to more consistently attending to, praising, and reinforcing appropriate behavior. In the second phase of treatment (parent-directed interaction), therapists focus on improving the child's compliance by setting behavioral limits and expectations. Therapists train parents to give only essential directions and commands, to make them clear and direct, maximizing chances for compliance by the child. Parents participating in PCIT traditionally learn a specific method of using time-out for dealing with noncompliance as well as other reliable strategies for managing difficult behavior. These strategies are designed to help caregivers avoid using physical power and to focus instead on using positive incentives and promoting children's emotional regulation.

INTERVENTIONS FOR MIDDLE CHILDHOOD

Interventions for children in middle childhood often incorporate thinking and reasoning into their protocols and move away from including parents in the child's treatment. Social behavior, attitudes, and perceptions of self and others become more important focuses of treatment. As in earlier years, negative emotions and emotional dysregulation also help indicate children's mental health status. The authors present an intervention commonly used with children in middle childhood and older: cognitive behavior therapy (CBT)[21] and a variation of CBT for traumatized children: trauma-focused cognitive behavioral therapy (TF-CBT).[22] Both have been rigorously researched.

CBT, originally called "cognitive therapy," was developed by Aaron Beck to treat depression.[21] Over the course of the past 5 decades, studies have shown it can be adapted to successfully treat children and adolescents with a wide variety of mental

How Parent-Child Interaction Therapy works

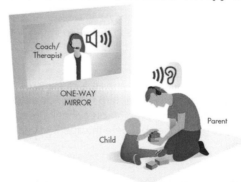

Fig. 3. PCIT therapy room and observation room diagram—how therapist coaching works with a "bug-in-the-ear" headset and earpiece.

health needs (eg, anxiety, obsessive compulsive disorder, bipolar disorder, eating disorders, personality disorders) and medical disorders (eg, chronic pain, migraines, inflammatory bowel disease).[23] A variation of this treatment, TF-CBT, received the highest ratings for demonstrating its effectiveness in reducing trauma symptoms.[24]

Cognitive Behavioral Therapy

Guiding principles
CBT is based on the idea that psychopathology arises from dysfunctional thinking and other problems in information processing. Depression and anxiety may arise from underlying negative beliefs about the self, other people, and the environment. Therefore, as illustrated by the graphic in **Fig. 4**, mental health problems can be resolved by targeting and adjusting thoughts, behaviors, and emotions.

Goals of treatment
The goals of CBT are to reduce mental health symptoms and relapse rates by identifying negative beliefs, perceptions, and thoughts and replace them with more constructive thinking, behavior, and emotional responses.

Strategies for achieving goals/procedures
Whether an individual has problems with anxiety, depression, or other mental health problems, therapeutic strategies for reducing symptoms In CBT are similar. Therapists identify patients' cognitive reactions and "automatic thoughts" and continue to refine their conceptualization of the patient's problems over the course of treatment. Because CBT aims to prevent relapse of symptoms, one of the goals is to educate patients about identifying new goals and responding to new problematic thoughts and behaviors as they arise, making positive adjustments. CBT requires a strong alliance between the therapist and patient to ensure active collaboration during treatment.

The course of treatment requires between 6 and 14 weekly structured sessions. Sessions include a check-in where the therapist assesses the patient's mood and reviews the "action plan" given at the prior session, which might include practicing strategies to replace certain negative thoughts with more realistic ones. Following this, the patient identifies the problems they want to work on that session. The therapist then evaluates thoughts, emotions, and behaviors surrounding the current problem. Collaboratively, they come up with an "action plan" for the coming week to handle

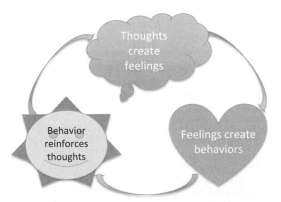

Fig. 4. The cognitive triangle—thoughts and memories trigger feelings and emotions, which drives us to take action. These actions or behaviors have consequences and meaning, which reinforce the original thoughts.

each problem the patient identifies. Finally, the patient gives the therapist feedback about the session and the "action plan" for the next week.

Trauma-focused Cognitive Behavioral Therapy

Guiding principles

Consistent with other CBT interventions, TF-CBT is based on the idea that processing and reframing thoughts about trauma, and implementing active strategies to avoid or minimize physiologic responses to stressors, improve functioning and reduces trauma symptoms.

Goals of treatment

TF-CBT aims to reduce trauma-related symptoms (eg, posttraumatic stress disorder [PTSD], depression, anxiety, and shame) in children and adolescents. TF-CBT also includes a component for nonoffending parents to help them support their child, decrease their own emotional distress, and enhance positive parenting.

Strategies for achieving goals

The strategies TF-CBT uses to achieve its treatment goals can be summarized by the acronym PRACTICE:

- *Psychoeducation* about the type of trauma the child has experienced, validating their reactions
- *Parenting module* to enhance positive parenting skills and improve strategies to manage children's behavior
- *Relaxation skills* to help control physiologic hyperarousal, like focused breathing or progressive muscle relaxation (for parents and children)
- *Affective modulation skills* to help children identify feelings, practice thought interruption, and enhance their use of positive self-talk
- *Cognitive processing* to help children and parents recognize connections between thoughts, feelings, and behaviors, and help change thoughts to be more accurate and helpful
- *Trauma narration* of the child's trauma experience, uncovering any cognitive distortions
- *In vivo desensitization* to help children overcome generalized avoidance of trauma reminders
- *Conjoint child-parent sessions* after the above components have been successfully completed
- *Enhancing safety* and future development for the child and parent

Accomplishing the PRACTICE protocol usually takes approximately 12 to 16 sessions lasting 60 to 90 minutes.

INTERVENTIONS FOR ADOLESCENTS

Two interventions often used with high-risk adolescents are described: dialectical behavior therapy (DBT)[25] and multisystemic therapy for child abuse and neglect (MSN-CAN).[26] Both interventions have a strong empirical foundation; both are interventions that have been adapted for treating adolescent clients with severe, unremitting, and complex mental health systems associated with child maltreatment. DBT has been shown to be effective in the treatment of mood disorders that often include suicidal behavior and self-harm[27] and with victims of sexual abuse.[28] MST-CAN addresses the referral behaviors plus key environmental risk factors that keep families coming through the revolving door of child protection.

Dialectical Behavior Therapy

Guiding principles

DBT[25] is based on the premise that acceptance and change occur through a dialectical process, in which the thesis (ie, clients' original beliefs) plus antithesis (adaptive alternatives) equal change. This dialectical change is enabled by clients' increased ability to tolerate distress, regulate emotions, improve interpersonal functioning, and increase mindfulness of themselves in their environment.

Goals of treatment

The overall goal of DBT is helping clients create "lives worth living," which involves achieving 4 distinct primary treatment objectives:

1. Increased control over behavior, increasing attention, and increasing distress tolerance
2. Improved emotional expression, reducing symptoms of PTSD
3. Improved problem-solving skills
4. Increased interpersonal connectedness

Strategies for achieving goals

DBT uses CBT-like behavioral techniques and cognitive restructuring and introduces the importance of mindfulness practice, validation, and principles of dialectical philosophy. The primary clinical tools used in DBT are diary cards, where the client records self-injurious and therapy-interfering behaviors throughout the week, and a functional analysis of sequences of behaviors (to increase mindfulness). Clients have weekly individual and group treatment sessions. During individual therapy, the therapist and patient work toward improving skill use. During group therapy, clients learn to use mindfulness skills, assertiveness skills for increasing interpersonal effectiveness, emotion regulation, and distress tolerance skills. Individual sessions are considered necessary to keep suicidal urges or uncontrolled emotional issues from disrupting group sessions, whereas the group sessions teach the skills unique to DBT and provide supervised opportunities for regulating emotions and behavior. Clients have telephone access to therapists 24 hours a day for help managing new skills and urgent problems. Therapists are required to participate in ongoing consultation team meetings to maintain or improve their own motivation. It takes approximately 1 year for clients to complete a typical course of treatment in DBT.

Multisystemic Therapy for Child Abuse and Neglect

Guiding principles

MST-CAN is a networked system of interventions based on a model that asserts that children are parts of various systems or "ecologies" (eg, school, family, parents) that they influence and that influence them. MST-CAN is guided by the belief that treatment must attend to the children's functioning in all of their social systems in order to be successful.

Goals of treatment

The overarching goals for MST-CAN are to keep families together safely by preventing placement out of the home, eliminating further incidents of maltreatment, and altering key factors that heighten maltreatment risk. As a strengths-based model, MST-CAN targets protective factors in children's social systems, particularly social support, and designs strategies to build upon them and use them as leverage for change. In cases where maltreatment has occurred, the MST team assesses risk factors and functioning across these systems and develops strategies to reduce risk (eg, parent mental health problems, housing, and employment problems) and improve child functioning (eg, aggressive behavior, depressive symptoms).

Strategies for achieving goals

The families referred to MST-CAN are those with multiple, serious clinical problems who have a child in the family who is between 6 and 17 years of age with a documented history of physical abuse or neglect within the last 180 days.

On average, 5 people per family are treated. For example, the parent may be treated for substance abuse, the grandmother for depression, and the child for behavioral problems at school. The team, consisting of 3 to 4 masters-level therapists, a case manager, and a consulting psychiatrist, works a flexible schedule seeing families at times that are convenient for them. Sessions may be during traditional work hours, at night, or on the weekend. The team operates a 24 hour per day, 7 days per week, with on-call rotation service to help families manage crises.

Most of the research-supported treatments used in MST-CAN are behavioral or cognitive-behavioral. For instance, therapists use cognitive behavioral treatments for anger management and behaviorally based family treatment for communication and problem-solving. Therapists use stress innoculation training[29] and prolonged exposure therapies[30] to reduce PTSD symptoms, and reinforcement-based treatment[31] to treat substance misuse.

DISCUSSION

In this article, the long-lasting effects of adverse events on children are described. The connection between attachment and the stress-response system, and the ways in which parenting and the family context continues to play a part in the way children respond to stress in their environment are described. The observable effects of these adverse events have been described: externalizing, disruptive behaviors in early years, social problems, school difficulties, and depression and other problems as children grew older (**Fig. 5**).

The evidence-based treatments that are described were selected because they represented the general type of service provided to children in that age group and because they had a strong evidence base. Interestingly, they all incorporated some strategy for improving emotional regulation and often targeted parenting strategies or family systems as mechanisms of change or methods for sustaining change.

The increasingly sophisticated literature describing the neurobiological effects of early adversity suggests that the stress response system may continue to play a part in undermining mental health throughout childhood and adolescence. The most effective treatments will likely include a component to help clients use active and cognitive strategies for controlling their responses to stress. In addition, early caregiving quality also appears to influence later interpersonal functioning, and the family system continues to support resilience. The most effective treatments for young children will also consider family systems and the parent-child relationship as key to future health.

The authors opted to take a more "meta" view of empirically based treatments for children with special needs, choosing different types and modalities of treatment delivery as representative interventions. Space limitations made it impossible to showcase all the excellent and promising interventions for children. For additional information about evidence-based treatments for children, the reader is directed to the California Evidence-Based Clearinghouse for Child Welfare (www.cebc4cw.org) for a nearly exhaustive list of available interventions. It is hoped that others will continue the work of examining mechanisms of effectiveness of evidence-based

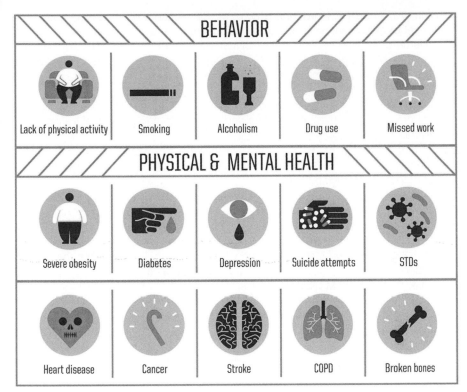

Fig. 5. The effects of ACEs. COPD, chronic obstructive pulmonary disease; STD, sexually transmitted disease.

treatments for maltreated children and to document the core components of effective mental health treatments.

ACKNOWLEDGMENTS

The authors would like to acknowledge the valuable contributions of Lindsay A. Forte, MS and Deanna K. Boys, MA in helping author this article.

REFERENCES

1. Perou R, Bitsko RH, Blumberg SJ, et al. Mental health surveillance among children—United States, 2005-2011. MMWR Surveill Summ 2013;62(Suppl 2):1–25.
2. Simpson GA, Cohen RA, Pastor PN, et al. Use of mental health services in the past 12 months by children aged 4–17 years: United States, 2005–2006. NCHS data brief, no 8. Hyattsville (MD): National Center for Health Statistics; 2008.
3. Cicchetti D, Lynch M. Toward an ecological/transactional model of community violence and child maltreatment: consequences for children's development. Psychiatry 1993;56:96–118.
4. Cicchetti D, Rogosch FA, Gunnar MR, et al. The differential impacts of early physical and sexual abuse and internalizing problems on daytime cortisol rhythm in school-aged children. Child Dev 2010;81:252–69.
5. McEwen B, Stellar E. Stress and the individual mechanisms leading to disease. Arch Intern Med 1993;153:2093–101.

6. Felitti VJ, Anda RF, Nordenberg D, et al. Relationship of childhood abuse and household dysfunction to many of the leading causes of death in adults: the adverse childhood experiences (ACE) study. Am J Prev Med 1998;14:245–58.

7. Gartstein M, Bridgett D, Dishion T, et al. Depressed mood and maternal report of child behavior problems: another look at the depression-distortion hypothesis. Dev Psychol 2009;30:149–60.

8. Goodman S, Gotlib I. Risk for psychopathology in the children of depressed mothers: a developmental model for understanding mechanisms of transmission. Psychol Rev 1999;60:458–90.

9. Bernard K, Dozier M, Bick J, et al. Intervening to enhance cortisol regulation among children at risk for neglect: results of a randomized clinical trial. Dev Psychopathol 2015;27(3):829–41.

10. Martorell GA, Bugental DB. Maternal variations in stress reactivity: implications for harsh parenting practices with very young children. J Fam Psychol 2006; 20(4):641–7.

11. Dube SR, Anda RF, Felitti VJ, et al. Childhood abuse, household dysfunction, and the risk of attempted suicide throughout the life span: findings from the adverse childhood experiences study. JAMA 2001;286:3089–96.

12. Pollak S, Messner M, Kistler D, et al. Development of perceptual expertise in emotion recognition. Cognition 2009;110:242–7.

13. Perlman SB, Kalish CW, Pollak SD. The role of maltreatment experience in children's understanding of the antecedents of emotion. Cogn Emot 2008;22(4): 651–70.

14. Deblinger E, Runyon MK. Understanding and treating feelings of shame in children who have experienced maltreatment. Child Maltreat 2005;10:364–76.

15. Chen P, Coccaro EF, Lee R, et al. Moderating effects of childhood maltreatment on associations between social information processing and adult aggression. Psychol Med 2012;4(6):1293–304.

16. Bolger K, Patterson C. Pathways from child maltreatment to internalizing problems: perceptions of control as mediators and moderators. Dev Psychopathol 2001;13(4):913–40.

17. Bernard K, Dozier M, Carlson E, et al. Enhancing attachment organization among maltreated children: results of a randomized clinical trial. Child Dev 2012;83(2): 623–36.

18. Lieberman AF, Weston D, Pawl J. Preventive intervention and outcome with anxiously attached dyads. Child Dev 1991;62:199–209.

19. Substance Abuse and Mental Health Services Administration (SAMHSA). Interventions for disruptive behavior disorders: evidence-based and promising practices. HHS Pub. No. SMA-11-4634. Rockville (MD): Center for Mental Health Services; SAMHSA; U.S. Department of Health and Human Services; 2011.

20. Eyberg S, Robinson EA. Parent-child interaction training: effects on family functioning. J Clin Child Psychol 1982;11(2):130–7.

21. Beck AT. Cognitive therapy: nature and relation to behavior therapy. Behav Ther 1970;1(2):184–200.

22. Cohen JA, Mannarino AP, Deblinger E. Treating trauma and traumatic grief in children and adolescents. New York: Guilford Press; 2006.

23. Beck JS. Cognitive behavior therapy, second edition: basics and beyond. New York: Guilford Press; 2011.

24. Mannarino AP, Cohen J, Deblinger E. Trauma-focused cognitive behavioral therapy. In: Timmer S, Urquiza A, editors. In evidence-based approaches for the

treatment of maltreated children: considering core components and treatment effectiveness. New York: Springer; 2014. p. 165–85.

25. Linehan MM. Skills training manual for treating borderline personality disorder. New York: Guilford Press; 1993.

26. Swenson CC, Schaeffer CM, Henggeler SW, et al. Multisystemic therapy for child abuse and neglect: a randomized effectiveness trial. J Fam Psychol 2010;24: 497–507.

27. Kliem S, Kröger C, Kossfelder J. Dialectical behavior therapy for borderline personality disorder: a meta-analysis using mixed-effects modeling. J Consult Clin Psychol 2010;78:936–51.

28. Decker SE, Naugle AE. DBT for sexual abuse survivors: current status and future directions. The Journal of Behavior Analysis of Offender and Victim Treatment and Prevention 2008;1(4):52–68.

29. Kilpatrick DG, Veronen LJ, Resick PA. Psychological sequelae to rape. In: Doleys DM, Meredith RL, editors. Behavioral medicine: assessment and treatment strategies. New York: Plenum Press; 1982. p. 473–97.

30. Foa EB, Rothbaum BO. Treating the trauma of rape: cognitive behavioral therapy for PTSD. New York: Guilford Press; 1998.

31. Tuten M, Jones HE, Schaeffer CM, et al. Reinforcement-based treatment (RBT): a practical guide for the behavioral treatment of drug addiction. Washington, DC: American Psychological Association; 2012.

Transitions in Health Care
What Can We Learn from Our Experience with Cystic Fibrosis

Natalie E. West, MD, MHS[a],*, Peter J. Mogayzel Jr, MD, PhD, MBA[b]

KEYWORDS

- Transition of health care • Cystic fibrosis • Pediatric medicine • Adult medicine
- Chronic disease

KEY POINTS

- Transition from pediatric to adult medical care can be a difficult process, particularly combined with the challenges of adolescence.
- Cystic fibrosis (CF) is an example of a chronic disease that has a growing adult population and has initiated transition care guidelines.
- The transition process should start early in adolescence with the focus each year concentrating on age-appropriate goals. Therefore, the individual is independent and ready for transfer to adult medical care by age 18 to 19 years.
- Elements of a successful transition for patients with CF include initiation of a multidisciplinary team, early transition program, transition meeting between health care providers, and transition clinic for patients.
- The elements of a successful transition that the CF community has identified can be extrapolated to help individuals with other chronic diseases.

INTRODUCTION

More than 500,000 adolescents with special health care needs in the United States reach adulthood each year.[1] These individuals have a wide variety of diseases, including cystic fibrosis (CF), sickle cell disease, congenital heart disease, diabetes, and neuromuscular disorders.[1] The improvement in survival for children with chronic diseases that arise in childhood has necessitated the development of transition programs to facilitate transfer of care from pediatric to adult care providers. The

Disclosure Statement: The authors have nothing to disclose.
a Division of Pulmonary and Critical Care Medicine, Johns Hopkins University, 1830 East Monument Street, 5th Floor, Baltimore, MD 21205, USA; b Department of Pediatrics, Cystic Fibrosis Center, Johns Hopkins Cystic Fibrosis Center, 200 North Wolfe Street, Rubenstein Child Health Building #3053, Baltimore, MD 21287-2533, USA
* Corresponding author.
E-mail address: nwest5@jhmi.edu

importance of developing a strong transition plan that ensures that "high-quality, developmentally appropriate health care services are available in an uninterrupted manner as the person moves from adolescence to adulthood" has been emphasized by a joint consensus statement by the American Academy of Pediatrics, Academy of Family Physicians, and American College of Physicians/American Society of Internal Medicine.[2]

Adolescence can be a challenging period, for both children and their families, and the addition of a chronic illness can affect normal development during this time. Similarly, the normal challenges of adolescence can adversely affect the health of an individual with a chronic illness.[3] For example, medication adherence often decreases as teenagers take more responsibility for their own care. Patients can be concerned over how their peers view their disease and may hide their need to take medications. Pediatric care providers can help their patients by being aware of the issues that can affect adolescents and their impact on their health, and by planning effective interventions to prevent some of these complications from occurring. Therefore, the carefully planned transition of young adults with a chronic disease from a pediatric medical care team to an adult medical care team should be an important priority.

Transition has been defined as "the purposeful, planned movement of adolescents and young adults with chronic physical and medical conditions from child-centered to adult-oriented health care programs."[1] Transfer is the actual point in time when the patient moves from pediatric to adult care providers. Transition should be a planned process over time, because a rapid transfer to a new adult medical team could be ineffective or even disastrous.[3] The danger of an abrupt transfer is the severing of important and solid relationships in the pediatric care team, with little to no assurance that appropriate adult care will be instituted.[3]

The transition of patients from pediatric to adult care should begin years before the actual transfer. In fact, some would say that the process of transition begins at diagnosis when prognosis and expectations are discussed. The process of transition involves education of both patient and family, assuring that the patient has an understanding of his or her disease, including the rationale for therapies and prognosis, and an assessment that the patient can independently manage therapies and navigate the health care system. Work, relationships, reproductive health issues, and family planning emerge as important issues at the time of transfer.[4] The transition of care is often made difficult because of the fear of losing long-standing relationships with pediatric caregivers as well as the fear of the new unknown adult caregiver. Other challenges include hesitance to be independent from parents, severity of illness, stability (recent exacerbations of illness that might delay transfer), emotional readiness of both the patient and the parent, longevity of care with the pediatric center, and emotional ties to providers. In addition, adult care practices may be different from previous experiences (eg, new treatments, new rules, new ways of treating infections, new faces [doctors, nurses, social worker, administrators, staff]), and new inpatient floors with all new nurses. Thus, assessing patient self-care readiness, adherence to medications, and psychosocial status is critical to ensuring a successful transfer.[4]

Transition Issues in Cystic Fibrosis

CF is the most common, life-shortening, genetic disorder of Caucasians. Abnormal electrolyte transport in epithelial cells leads to a multisystem disorder characterized by significant sinus and pulmonary disease, pancreatic insufficiency, elevated sweat chloride, and male infertility.[5] Individuals with CF develop progressive airways obstruction characterized by abnormal mucus, chronic endobronchial infection, and inflammation. Pulmonary exacerbations, characterized by increased cough and/or sputum production, are the hallmark of the disease and occur frequently in individuals with CF and are associated with loss of lung function, worsened quality of life, and decreased survival.[3,6–11] Most CF individuals die from pulmonary complications, and thus, a major goal of CF treatment is slowing the progression of lung disease.[5,12,13] Individuals with CF are prescribed a complex daily regimen of airway clearance and inhaled medications to modify the abnormal mucus and minimize infection. In addition, more intense therapies, including hospitalization, are often required to treat pulmonary exacerbations.

Fortunately, individuals with CF are living longer, because there has been significant improvement in survival over the past 40 years.[3,11] In the 1950s, individuals survived to a median age of 5. The median predicted survival of only 16 years in 1970 is now up to 39.3 years (**Fig. 1**).[11] This increase in survival is largely due to improvements in therapies for CF, including inhaled medications, antibiotics, pancreatic enzymes, and airway clearance. In addition, the dramatic increase in median survival in CF has resulted in a significant growth in the number of individuals with CF more than 18 years old (adults), with 50% of individuals being 18 years or older (**Fig. 2**).[11]

The dramatic improvement in survival and the increasing number of individuals reaching adulthood have necessitated the development of adult CF care programs. In fact, by the end of 2000, CF centers that cared for 40 or more adults were required to have separate pediatric and adult programs staffed by care teams with age-appropriate training to maintain CF Foundation accreditation.[14] This mandate also emphasized developing a process to transition to adult care and developing evidence-based clinical care guidelines.

The timing of transfer to adult CF care often coincides with changes associated with adolescence when lung function may be declining and treatment burden increasing.[15] Adults with CF have more obstacles to hurdle, including worsening lung function, often requiring intravenous antibiotics and hospitalizations (**Fig. 3**).[11] Complications also become more prevalent in adulthood, specifically bone disease, CF-related diabetes, depression, and arthritis (**Fig. 4**).[16] Therefore, not only does the patient have to go through transition to a new medical team but also they also may have to face new diagnoses and additional medications and treatments requiring more effort, time, and dedication.

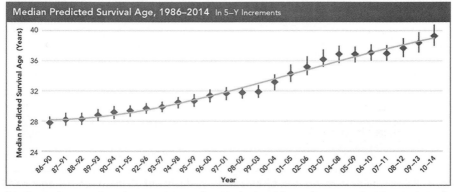

Fig. 1. Median predicted survival age of individuals with CF. (*From* Cystic Fibrosis Foundation Patient Registry. 2014 Annual Data Report. Bethesda, Maryland; © 2015 Cystic Fibrosis Foundation.)

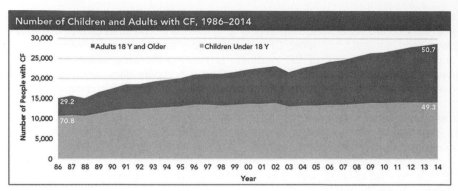

Fig. 2. The number of children and adults with CF. (*From* Cystic Fibrosis Foundation Patient Registry. 2014 Annual Data Report. Bethesda, Maryland; © 2015 Cystic Fibrosis Foundation.)

What We Can Learn from Cystic Fibrosis?

CF is an example of a chronic disease whereby much effort has been put into implementing models to improve transition from pediatric care to adult care. The CF Foundation, a nonprofit organization that supports CF research and clinical care, made the successful transition of pediatric patients to adult caregivers a critical part of its mission. The CF Foundation was established in 1955 and now accredits ~120 CF centers. Beyond advocating transition, the CF Foundation developed Adult Care Consensus Guidelines to provide goals and help standardize care.[3] In addition, when it became clear that there were an inadequate number of appropriately trained adult providers, the CF Foundation supported the training of additional providers. Perhaps the most important lesson from the CF experience is that developing a transition program from pediatric to adult care is critically important and does not develop without committed individuals. However, the success of the transition process also

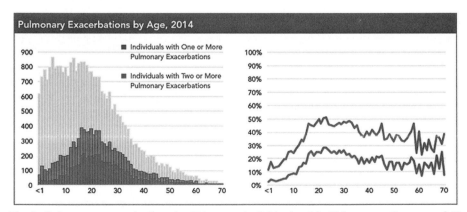

Fig. 3. Pulmonary exacerbations in CF by age. Individuals with CF between the ages of 15 and 30 are more likely to experience an exacerbation each year, compared with other age groups. (*From* Cystic Fibrosis Foundation Patient Registry. 2014 Annual Data Report. Bethesda, Maryland; © 2015 Cystic Fibrosis Foundation.)

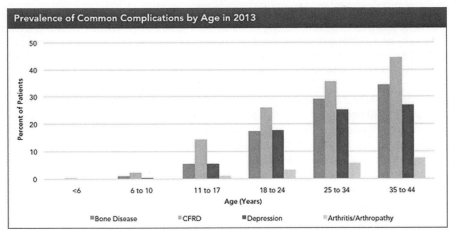

Fig. 4. Prevalence of common CF complications by age. (*From* Cystic Fibrosis Foundation Patient Registry. 2014 Annual Data Report. Bethesda, Maryland; © 2015 Cystic Fibrosis Foundation.)

depends on making sure that there are an adequate number of appropriately trained adult care providers.

There are several principles that care providers of individuals with CF have adopted that can be applied generally to other chronic diseases that affect individuals in both young and older ages. There must be commitment by both the pediatric and the adult teams to ensure frequent communication and shared responsibility to make a transition program successful for their patients. Transition should be coordinated and gradual, addressing concerns of both the patient and his or her parents, promoting independence and education, and providing flexibility to address concerns of the individual being transitioned.[15]

The model of a multidisciplinary team providing care for individuals with CF has been established in pediatric care centers and also has been incorporated into the care of adults with CF.[3] Ideally, these care teams include physicians, nurses, dieticians, respiratory therapists, physical therapists, social workers, and psychologists. In an outpatient clinic visit, the patient has the opportunity to meet with several members of this team, depending on their current issues. These same team members are often also involved in the inpatient setting, providing continuity. As individuals age into adulthood, there is generally a higher incidence of more severe pulmonary disease, higher prevalence of CF-related diabetes, and more complex financial and psychosocial issues.[3] Therefore, the expertise of this multidisciplinary team becomes necessary, and there is a consensus that a multidisciplinary team with training in adult CF should care for these patients. This model could be helpful in other chronic illnesses, such as sickle cell disease and congenital heart disease.

In 1999, Johns Hopkins Hospital developed an Adult CF Program and transitioned 80 adults from the pediatric center over 5 months.[17] This allowed for an evaluation of the transition process as well as assessment of the concerns of patients transitioning from the pediatric center to the adult center. Sixty patients and their parents filled out a pretransition survey 3 months before transfer and an after-transition interview 8 to 12 months after transfer.[17] Survey questions were used to identify concerns individuals had about transitioning as well as expectations individuals had for an adult CF program. Results showed that individuals with CF had significant concerns about potential exposure to infection, having to leave their previous physician, meeting a new care team, and a potential decrease in the quality of medical care. After the transition, there was a statistically significant decrease in all areas except for concerns about potential exposure to infection and being admitted to the adult hospital (**Fig. 5**).[17] In particular, concerns about leaving behind a previous physician and meeting a new team dropped to "no concern" levels.[17] Of the 52 patients who completed the pretransition survey, 30 had met the adult team in the pediatric clinic before they completed the survey. In those patients who had met the adult team, their responses demonstrated statistically significant lower levels of concern (compared with those patients who had not met the adult team) in all areas, particularly in levels of concern about leaving previous physicians and a potential decline in quality of care (**Fig. 6**).[17] Overall, young adults with CF reported satisfaction in the transfer process when they were able to meet with both the pediatric and the adult teams together, before their first appointment with the adult team.[3,17] Hence, most CF centers have worked to establish transition clinics where pediatric and adult care providers communicate about each patient transitioning, and members of the adult care team meet with the patient along with the pediatric team.

In 2008, more than 85% of individuals with CF were followed by CF Foundation accredited centers, indicating that research data from these centers would represent a comprehensive view of the transition process in the CF community.[1] Therefore, McLaughlin and colleagues[1] conducted a survey of the 195 CF care programs in the United States on transition practices. Transition activities were accessed in 7 functional domains: patient preparation, patient readiness assessment, coordination of

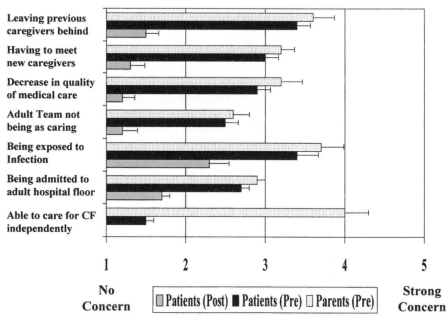

Fig. 5. Areas of concern before and after transition of care from pediatric to adult care. Groups include 38 parents pretransition (*stippled bar*), 52 patients pretransition (*black bar*), and 60 patients after transition (*gray bar*). (*From* Boyle MP, Farukhi Z, Nosky ML. Strategies for improving transition to adult cystic fibrosis care, based on patient and parent views. Pediatr Pulmonol 2001;32(6):431; with permission.)

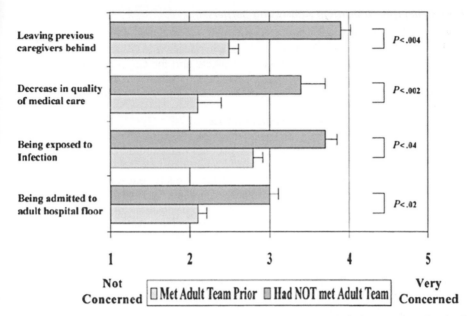

Fig. 6. Effect of meeting adult team before transition. Groups included 22 patients that had not met the adult team before transition and 30 patients who had met the adult team before transition. Previous exposure to the adult team significantly reduced the level of concern in all areas. (*From* Boyle MP, Farukhi Z, Nosky ML. Strategies for improving transition to adult cystic fibrosis care, based on patient and parent views. Pediatr Pulmonol 2001;32(6):432; with permission.)

services and benefits, information transfer (communication of medical summary), primary and preventative health care, patient follow-up and program evaluation, and transition program self-evaluation. Responses were received from 87% of CF Foundation–accredited centers. Results showed that the initial discussion of transition occurred at median age of 17 years (range "time from diagnosis" to 25 years). Transfer of care took place at a median age of 19 years (range 14–30).[1] More than 80% of programs reported having a discussion involving transition of a patient at a pediatric care team meeting, yet only one-third of programs had the adult care provider present for those meetings.[1] This study had several key findings including that the process of transition was beginning late (at 17 years), which left little time to adequately prepare the patient and their families for transfer. Strengths of the existent transition process at that time included high involvement with counseling on substance abuse, smoking, and dietary behavior. However, only half of the centers focused on the ability to list medications, taking medications without being reminded, and being able to contact caregiver or insurance independently.[1] Almost half of the programs reported rarely preparing a medical summary before transfer. The recognition that the transition process in CF was not acceptable led to the recommendations mentioned in later discussion, and in particular, the development of a list of self-management skills per age group that the CF Foundation could endorse. Specifically, the goals were to introduce the transition at an earlier age, aim to help the individual with CF develop self-management skills, and establish nationally recognized age-specific goals for people transitioning to adult care.[1]

How to Improve Transition: Addressing Barriers

Over the last 20 years, the CF Care Center Network has developed adult CF programs to augment pediatric programs to provide care to people with CF across the age spectrum. Research and quality improvement projects and the CF center have identified areas that can make transition a success.[14] Although further work is still needed, there are several processes that have been shown to be beneficial in transition.

Make transition to adult care a gradual process

A successful transition to adult care should not begin at age 18 to 21. It can begin as early as age 13 or earlier.[18,19] Transition is a process that occurs over years, and transfer is the actual point in which the transfer to adult care takes place. The initiation of age-appropriate responsibilities can be introduced each year, and the initial steps can be simple at first. For instance, an initial goal at age 12 could be patients knowing the names of their medications and why they are using them. At age 13, the child should be able to talk about the amount of medication they take and when they should be taking them each day. At age 14, the responsibility of talking directly with their pediatrician during clinic visits with occasional input from parents should be a reachable goal. The adolescent can gradually be given more responsibility for self-care and decision making and should be seen alone in clinic. Therefore, by the age of 18, the child should know enough about their chronic disease but also feel comfortable talking to their physician on their own. They should be able to contact their physicians with changes in health, schedule appointments, and refill prescriptions. A more intense preparation should take place the year before transfer is planned, which may include tours of the adult inpatient and outpatient centers and meeting members of the adult team. Taking these gradual steps over the years will lead to a successful transition when it becomes time to transition to an adult medical team. **Table 1** lists specific CF age-specific recommendations.[18,19]

Remember that parents are going through a transition as well

It may be easy to only concentrate on the process of guiding a child through transition, and the parent-child relationship and the parent-physician relationship are forgotten.[18] It can be a hard adjustment on a parent when a pediatrician or adult physician asks to see their child alone. Supporting the parent through this process is beneficial as well, and the parents need to be reminded that the physician is trying to help their child grow up.

Work together to improve transition

The pediatric and adult teams should have a formal transfer meeting before transfer date. This formal transfer meeting includes the pediatric team (physicians, nurses, social worker, and so forth) meeting with the same individuals from the adult team. This meeting serves as a way to communicate to each patient who is ready to transfer, and what their specific issues might be. The pediatric team should create a medical summary for all transitioning patients nearing readiness for transfer. A peer-to-peer transition might be helpful (pediatric physician specifically talks to adult physician, and similar for nurse to nurse, social worker to social worker communication), because different concerns are relevant from each member of the team. After this meeting, the adult care team should attend a transition clinic visit with the patient. This transition clinic visit serves as their last pediatric visit, and a chance to meet a few members of the adult medical team on familiar ground. Generally, this should include a physician, nurse, and/or social worker. The intent of this clinic visit is not to discuss medical issues and plans on treating the patient, but rather it is to introduce how the adult center

Table 1
Age-appropriate transition goals of individuals with cystic fibrosis

	12 y	13–14 y	15–16 y	17–18 y	19–21 y
Transition goals	Describe what CF is	List medications, amounts, and times when taken	Become better at recognizing symptoms and describing them	Contact CF caregivers directly to discuss changes in health	Contact CF caregivers directly to discuss changes in health
	Name medications and reasons for taking them	Answer questions independently in clinic	Describe choices about smoking and drinking and effect on health	Schedule appointments and tests	Schedule appointments and tests
	Take enzymes	Recognize changes in symptoms and describe them	Be aware of clinic and test appointment dates	Refill prescriptions	Refill prescriptions
	Remember to do airway clearance	Do airway clearance without help	Be aware of medication supply and need for refills	Maintaining own equipment	Learn details about insurance coverage

Data from Boyle MP. Transitioning to adult care: a transition for parents as well! Article on MyCysticFibrosis.com Web site. 2007; and Boyle MP, Mogayzel PJ. Partnering for care: help your adult CF center help you thrive. 2010. Available at: https://www.cff.org/PDF-archive/partnering-for-care-slides–partnering-as-an-adult-with-CF/.

works, meet friendly faces, and reassure the patient and their family they will continue to be well taken care of. The Adult CF Care Consensus recommends CF centers designate a coordinator to help the patient through the transfer process (scheduling appointments with the adult center, helping with insurance issues, and addressing psychosocial issues that may come up).[3]

At the first adult clinic visit, this introduction should continue, with introduction of the rest of the team members. Any changes in medical treatment should be made gradually, over several visits, to avoid confusion and the perception that there is disagreement on previous care. The CF Foundation guidelines recommend clinic visits once every 3 months. If an individual has a more severe illness that is complicated, they could be seen once a month for the first several months so that they become comfortable with the new adult team, and the adult caregivers have the opportunity to learn their medical and social issues efficiently.

Potential Resources

The CF Transition Advisory Council and Gilead Sciences, Inc, have developed CF R.I.S.E., which stands for Responsibility, Independence, Self-Care, Education.[20] This program was developed to provide CF care teams with patient materials to help manage the transition and transfer process. CF R.I.S.E. comprises a series of CF education and skills assessments on various topics designed to identify areas that need more focus and support, allowing the patient and care team to work together to develop a personalized and focused plan. Knowledge assessments ensure that conversations are occurring about all areas of CF care. In this way, education deficits are discovered that can be corrected.

SUMMARY

Transition from pediatric care to adult care in the setting of a chronic disease can be challenging, and it is important to have a successful health care transition program in place. Lessons learned from the care of people with CF have identified several factors that are associated with successful transition programs, including buy-in from both the pediatric and the adult teams, creation of a transition program that begins early in adolescence, establishment of a transition meeting for pediatric and adult providers to discuss individual patients, and creating a transition clinic or other venue where members of the adult team can meet patients and families before the actual transfer of care.

REFERENCES

1. McLaughlin SE, Diener-West M, Indurkhya A, et al. Improving transition from pediatric to adult cystic fibrosis care: lessons from a national survey of current practices. Pediatrics 2008;121(5):e1160–6.
2. American Academy of Pediatrics, American Academy of Family Physicians, American College of Physicians, et al, Transitions Clinical Report Authoring Group. Supporting the health care transition from adolescence to adulthood in the medical home. Pediatrics 2011;128(1):182–200.
3. Yankaskas JR, Marshall BC, Sufian B, et al. Cystic fibrosis adult care: consensus conference report. Chest 2004;125(Suppl 1):1S–39S.
4. Okumura MJ, Kleinhenz ME. Cystic fibrosis transitions of care: lessons learned and future directions for cystic fibrosis. Clin Chest Med 2016;37(1):119–26.
5. Boyle MP. Adult cystic fibrosis. JAMA 2007;298(15):1787–93.

6. Sanders DB, Hoffman LR, Emerson J, et al. Return of FEV1 after pulmonary exacerbation in children with cystic fibrosis. Pediatr Pulmonol 2010;45(2):127–34.
7. Liou TG, Adler FR, Fitzsimmons SC, et al. Predictive 5-year survivorship model of cystic fibrosis. Am J Epidemiol 2001;153(4):345–52.
8. Mayer-Hamblett N, Rosenfeld M, Emerson J, et al. Developing cystic fibrosis lung transplant referral criteria using predictors of 2-year mortality. Am J Respir Crit Care Med 2002;166(12 Pt 1):1550–5.
9. Emerson J, Rosenfeld M, McNamara S, et al. Pseudomonas aeruginosa and other predictors of mortality and morbidity in young children with cystic fibrosis. Pediatr Pulmonol 2002;34(2):91–100.
10. Ellaffi M, Vinsonneau C, Coste J, et al. One-year outcome after severe pulmonary exacerbation in adults with cystic fibrosis. Am J Respir Crit Care Med 2005; 171(2):158–64.
11. Cystic Fibrosis Foundation. Cystic fibrosis foundation patient registry, 2014 annual data report. Bethesda (MD): Cystic Fibrosis Foundation; 2015.
12. Flume PA, O'Sullivan BP, Robinson KA, et al. Cystic fibrosis pulmonary guidelines: chronic medications for maintenance of lung health. Am J Respir Crit Care Med 2007;176(10):957–69.
13. Flume PA, Mogayzel PJ Jr, Robinson KA, et al. Cystic fibrosis pulmonary guidelines: treatment of pulmonary exacerbations. Am J Respir Crit Care Med 2009; 180(9):802–8.
14. Mogayzel PJ Jr, Dunitz J, Marrow LC, et al. Improving chronic care delivery and outcomes: the impact of the cystic fibrosis care center network. BMJ Qual Saf 2014;23(Suppl 1):i3–8.
15. Tuchman LK, Schwartz LA, Sawicki GS, et al. Cystic fibrosis and transition to adult medical care. Pediatrics 2010;125(3):566–73.
16. Cystic Fibrosis Foundation. Cystic fibrosis foundation patient registry, 2013 annual data report. Bethesda (MD): Cystic fibrosis foundation; 2014.
17. Boyle MP, Farukhi Z, Nosky ML. Strategies for improving transition to adult cystic fibrosis care, based on patient and parent views. Pediatr Pulmonol 2001;32(6): 428–36.
18. Boyle MP. Transitioning to adult care: a transition for parents as well! Article on MyCysticFibrosis.com website. 2007.
19. Boyle MP, Mogayzel PJ. Partnering for care: help your adult CF center help you thrive. 2010. Available at: https://www.cff.org/PDF-archive/partnering-for-care-slides–partnering-as-an-adult-with-CF/.
20. Baker AM, Riekert KA, Sawicki GS, et al. CF RISE: implementing a clinic-based transition program. Pediatr Allergy Immunol Pulmonol 2015;28(4):250–4.

Integrating Pediatric Palliative Care into the School and Community

Kathleen G. Davis, PhD, MSEd

KEYWORDS

- Pediatric palliative care • Chronic illness • Quality of life • School • Transition
- Life-threatening • Life-limiting • Hospice

KEY POINTS

- Common terminology and definitions are needed to ensure a uniform language is used when developing comprehensive pediatric palliative care (CPPC) for children in need of the services and their family members.
- CPPC addresses the physical, psychological, social or emotional, and spiritual needs of children with complex chronic conditions, including some children with special health care needs.
- CPPC should occur at school, worship, athletics, clubs, and organizations where children develop healthy physical, psychological, social or emotional, and spiritual selves.
- Education and civil rights legislation provide a foundation for CPPC services in schools and community settings.
- When a child has an out-of-hospital do-not-resuscitate (OOH DNAR) order, heath care providers (HCPs) should partner with schools to provide support to the child and family, as well as to school professionals, to ensure a positive outcome for all parties. The development of CPPC may aid in enhancing communication between HCPs, families, and schools during the time when an OOH DNAR decision is being considered.

INTRODUCTION

Palliative care is patient and family-centered care that optimizes quality of life by anticipating, preventing, and treating suffering. The initiation of palliative care increasingly begins at diagnosis and continues throughout the illness trajectory.[1] Pediatric palliative care (PPC) is provided to children ranging in age from prenatal to young adult or older when receiving treatment of a pediatric diagnosis.[2] Most PPC is provided in a hospital setting; however, community-based PPC (CBPPC) programs are an integral component of assuring access to PPC for children with life-threatening illnesses when provided along with curative or life-prolonging treatment.[3,4]

Disclosure Statement: The author has nothing to disclose.
Department of Pediatrics, University of Kansas Medical Center, 3901 Rainbow Boulevard, MS4004, Kansas City, KS 66060, USA
E-mail address: kdavis2@kumc.edu

Pediatr Clin N Am 63 (2016) 899–911
http://dx.doi.org/10.1016/j.pcl.2016.06.013
0031-3955/16/$ – see front matter © 2016 Elsevier Inc. All rights reserved.

Children are dynamic beings who are learning, growing, and developing along a continuum that leads to self-awareness, self-advocacy, and competencies that enable the youngster to become a functional adult. Seriously ill children arrive to PPC at a point along that continuum of development and are very different from adults with serious illnesses. Children have not yet learned to cope with adversity, identified sources of support during a crisis, nor can they answer the question "Who am I?" Children may have encountered serious illness since birth, gradually entered into serious illness, or been thrust suddenly into the chaos. In any case, the focus quickly becomes the child's diagnosis and related challenges; however, that does not halt the child's movement along the developmental continuum as she or he continues to grow, change, and learn about herself or himself and the world. Throughout even the most serious of illnesses, the child continues to be a child and possesses all of the developmental, social, emotional, and spiritual needs of a child. To be effective, PPC must address the child's needs on a developmentally appropriate level for that individual child and provide services in the places where the child lives, learns, grows, and develops. Typically, that place is not the hospital. Rather, it is the child's natural environments of home, school, worship, play, friends, and other interactive activities.

Currently, there is a zeitgeist in our culture that presents an opportunity to change the way PPC is provided to children. Two generations ago, children with serious diagnoses lived in institutions, received minimal medical care, and did not attend school. For example, children with muscular dystrophy, cystic fibrosis,[5] or spina bifida[6] lived only into adolescence, whereas those with cerebral palsy or other neurologic or developmental disabilities were often institutionalized.[7] Today, many of those same youngsters are living into their 20s, 30s, and beyond. Medications, ventriculoperitoneal shunts, central venous access lines, gastrostomy tubes, and ventilators have increased the life expectancy of children with neuromuscular disorders.[8] Care in neonatal intensive care units has improved survival of premature infants[9] and infants with chronic heart or lung conditions, genetic disorders, or birth defects.[10] As children with serious illnesses are often living longer, schools, athletic teams, places of worship, and other venues are developing an understanding of the needs of these children. Thus, participating in school, athletics, and worship are viable options.

With increased survival come unavoidable consequences of significant disability and medical, educational, psychological, social, and spiritual challenges. More children are surviving, resulting in more children who need PPC. These PPC programs should provide coordinated, efficient, and cost-effective care.[11] Health care has opened the doors for seriously ill children to gain entry into activities. Therefore, the interdisciplinary PPC team is called on, in collaboration with adults in the child's natural environments, to engage a broad team of providers to provide a new definition of PPC: comprehensive PPC (CPPC).

This article considers the possibility of developing strong alliances and partnerships between hospitals, CBPPC, schools, athletic teams, places of worship, and other community-based organizations. Partnerships will result in increased knowledge for all caregivers, thus enabling children to have the opportunity to address physical, psychological, social or emotional, and spiritual needs in all of the natural environments where they live, learn, grow, and develop.

SPEAKING THE SAME LANGUAGE

In the interest of developing CPPC services provided across a child's natural environments, it is imperative that all stakeholders use consistent terminology to define the children and the services they will receive. Currently, heath care providers (HCPs) use terminology that is often unfamiliar to other professions. Other stakeholders may not yet have an awareness of PPC or their role in providing it. As groups work to develop a foundation for CPPC, an initial time investment will be required to identify and teach shared terminology, as well as the essential components of CPPC as it pertains to the psychological, social or emotional, and spiritual needs of the child and family. Uniformity in key terms will ensure that individuals from each profession are operating from the same conceptual base and can work collaboratively to provide comprehensive care.

PEDIATRIC PALLIATIVE CARE AND PEDIATRIC HOSPICE CARE

A greater number of infants, children, and adolescents (collectively referred to as children for the remainder of this article) receive both PPC and pediatric hospice care (PHC) than ever before. Although the terms palliative and hospice are often used synonymously, the meanings of these 2 models of care are actually quite different. Palliative care suggests a strong focus on the child's quality of life and may be provided to the child for months or years either as the main focus of care or, when appropriate, along with concurrent disease-modifying therapy.[2] The focus of PPC is on quality of life and enabling the young person to live as productive a life as possible despite the existence of a serious illness.

Conversely, PHC is a program and philosophy of care for children facing a life-limiting illness or condition who have a life expectancy of months, not years, and includes expert medical care, pain management, and psychological, social, and spiritual support expressly tailored to the patient's and family's needs and wishes. Hospice focuses on caring, not curing.[2]

Most definitions of PPC emphasize referral early in a child's disease trajectory and a focus on quality of life. The World Health Organization defines palliative care as

- The active total care of patients whose disease is not responsive to curative treatment. Control of pain, of other symptoms, and of psychological, social, and spiritual problems is paramount. The goal of palliative care is achievement of the best quality of life for patients and their families.[12]

The American Academy of Pediatrics (AAP) definition includes the following key points:

- PPC-PHC should be provided as collaborative integrated multimodal care, including cure-seeking, life-prolonging (when in the child's best interest), comfort-enhancing, and quality-of-life enriching modes of care.
- Psychological, spiritual, and social support for the family.
- Collaboration is essential. Patient, parents, other involved extended family members and friends, schools, parental employers, and all involved members of the primary and specialty health care team must collaborate to effectively meet the needs of patients.
- For all patients, high-quality PPC-PHC should routinely prevent and treat distressing symptoms, such as pain, nausea, or anxiety, and seek to maximize quality of life, which may entail various interventions, depending on the patient's specific goals.
- PPC consultations can occur throughout the child's illness experience, including at initial diagnosis, when the goals of care are focused on cure.
- PPC-PHC should be integrated throughout the illness course, providing interventions to support the goals of care, which often shift over time.[13]

Attempts to describe the specific population of children who receive PPC services in the United States have been inconsistent. Ages that are included in PPC are reported with different parameters. For example, most community and hospital PPC programs serve children up to age 19 years but some hospitals continue care to age 21 years or beyond. National Hospice and Palliative Care Organization's Standards of Practice for Pediatric Palliative/Hospice Care defines pediatrics as "for infants through young adults."[14] The adolescent and young adult population is defined by the National Cancer Institute as patients from 15 to 39 years of age.[15]

Other attempts to identify eligible children focus on prognoses referring to those who will die, those who may die, those with life-limiting or life-threatening diagnoses, and children who are terminally ill. The literature reports difficulty with prognostication identifying "unrealistic physician and/or parental prognostic expectations may be leading to inappropriate treatment goals"[16] and "We often do not know how long the patient may live or even whether he or she will survive the illness."[17] Thus, prognoses may not be reliable criteria for children in need of PPC.

Specific diagnoses that suggest children's eligibility for PPC may be the method with the greatest efficacy. The Center to Advance Palliative Care offers the Pediatric Palliative Care Referral Criteria[18] that identify diagnoses that should receive an automatic consult, as well as those diagnoses that suggest a palliative care referral. Chronic complex condition (CCC) is a broad descriptive category of specific diagnoses that identify many, if not most, children who receive PPC and sometimes PHC. The health care literature first described CCC as

- Any medical condition that can be reasonably expected to last at least 12 months (unless death intervenes) and to involve either several different organ systems or a single system severely enough to require specialty pediatric care and probably some period of hospitalization in a tertiary care center.[19]

The original definition of CCC identified 9 diagnostic categories, including cardiovascular, respiratory, neuromuscular, renal, gastrointestinal, hematologic or immunologic, metabolic, other congenital or genetic, and malignancy. The 2014 update added the category of premature and neonatal conditions. The update, which also addresses changes in the *International Classification of Diseases*, 10th revision, includes a domain of complexity arising from dependence on medical technology (devices), and a domain indicating the child has been the recipient of a transplant.[11]

Regardless of what method of eligibility is used, some children do not ever receive a timely referral to PPC. Data from a 2001 study by the Children's International Project on Palliative/Hospice Services estimated that on any given day 5000 children with CCCs were in the last 6 months of life and another 8600 children would be eligible for palliative care services. In addition, only 5000 of the 53,000 children who died that year received hospice services and usually only for a brief period of time.[20] A uniform definition would likely ensure that more children in need of PPC would be identified and, thus, receive referrals for care.

EDUCATION DEFINITIONS

It is anticipated that schools would be primary partners to HCPs in providing CPPC because children typically spend 7 to 8 hours a day in school. HCPs may benefit from understanding the terminology and reference point from which educators join the discussion.

In 1995, the Department of Health and Human Services Maternal and Child Health Bureau defined children with special health care needs as those

- Who have or are at increased risk of developing a chronic physical, developmental, behavioral, or emotional condition and who also require health and related services of a type or amount beyond that usually required by childhood conditions.[21]

This definition is commonly used in schools to describe students with serious chronic health conditions, 27% of whom have a condition or conditions that affect their activities usually, always, or a great deal.[22]

The 2009 to 2010 National Survey of Children with Special Health Care Needs (CSHCN; Chartbook 2013) indicates that

- Fifteen percent of children younger than 18 years of age in the United States, or more than 11 million children, have special health care needs.
- One in 4 households with children has at least 1 child with a special health care need.
- These health care needs include cystic fibrosis, asthma, diabetes, food allergy, sickle cell disease, juvenile idiopathic arthritis, genetic disorders, spina bifida, neuromuscular diseases, epilepsy, congenital heart diseases, trauma-related injury, and human immunodeficiency syndrome, as well as disorders of speech, language, learning, and behavior.
- Literature regarding CSHCN frequently refers to the existence of "limitation of function or activity."[23]

CSHCN is consistent with criteria used by schools to identify students who have a physical or health disability significant enough to result in special education services or accommodations to enable them to access educational and extracurricular activities. There are significant similarities between the categories of CCC and CSHCN. Both definitions

- Identify the existence of a serious chronic health condition
- Acknowledge the child's increased need for hospitalization or increased frequency of health care services
- Acknowledge that the number of children in the category is increasing
- Suggest an impact on the child's functional ability
- Includes children who may not have survived into childhood or adolescence if born a generation sooner.

There is a natural juncture for collaboration between health care and education in service delivery, research, resources to support the child and family, and broader advocacy and policy issues. Children with CCCs are already commonly identified as those in need of PPC and the terminology often appears in the health care literature. The similarities between CCC and CSHCN suggest the transition to using CCC may be easy for educators, whereas other collaborative partners do not routinely use this term to refer to children with serious health conditions. Therefore, CCC is used in this discussion and suggested for use in referring to the target population of children who could benefit from CPPC in all natural environments.

LEGISLATION AFFECTING EDUCATION OF CHILDREN WITH COMPLEX CHRONIC CONDITIONS

The history of education for students with serious health conditions is very brief. Compulsory education for children without disabilities was not introduced until the late nineteenth century and nearly a century later children with disabilities enjoyed the right to attend school. A few private and/or residential programs existed with no oversight regarding quality and availability of programs. Good programs were rare, difficult to access, and great variability existed between and within states. For most children with disabilities, special education programs were simply not available.[24]

The 1975 enactment of Public Law 94 to 142, later renamed the Individuals with Disabilities Education Act (IDEA), entitled all children, regardless of disability or special needs, to a free and appropriate public education at no cost to parents.[25] However, eligibility for special education is a process and to be eligible for special education services the child must have 1 of 13 specific categories of special needs, as well as have difficulty learning as a result of the disability. An assessment, using a variety of empirically based learning strategies, is conducted in the general education classroom by several professionals and may take several months. If none of those approaches to teaching are found to be successful, the student is determined to be in need of special education, or "specially designed instruction to meet the unique needs of the learner."[26]

Children who do not qualify for special education under IDEA may be protected under civil rights legislation in the form of Section 504 of the Rehabilitation Act of 1973, which provides accommodations and modifications at school. A 504 Plan provides accommodations and modifications to enable the learner to access all components of the school curriculum. Section 504 is designed to provide accommodations that will level the playing field for the individual with a disability; however, it does not provide special education.[27]

CHILD AND FAMILY NEEDS

Children play, learn, grow, and develop in a variety of locations, including home, school, places of worship, art, dance and music classes, and athletic teams. Even the sickest of children do not typically spend most of their time in a medical setting. Nonetheless, the model of PPC is typically purely medical with the HCP focusing on the physical, psychological, social, emotional, and spiritual well-being of the child at the hospital or home. To address the comprehensive needs of the child and family, a PPC program must extend beyond the walls of the hospice, hospital, or the child's home and into the world of the child. Many professionals are already providing care that addresses the child and family's psychosocial and spiritual well-being at school, at worship, and in other community settings.

Children with CCCs live at the crossroad of medicine and normal childhood. A child's self-concept is threatened by growing up with a serious diagnosis or by the knowledge that they may die as a result of their diagnosis. Parents worry about their ill child, the healthy siblings, financial concerns, maintaining their employment, and much more. Siblings may feel lost, angry, sad, or a host of other emotions that may be difficult for them to understand. The needs of the child, parents, siblings, peers, and the community bear consideration when palliative care is provided.

Children with CCCs require exquisite case management and effective collaboration between the professionals who care for them in the hospital, clinic, home, school, and various community settings. With appropriate PPC, children with CCCs may continue to see themselves as students, soccer players, artists, and friends rather than solely as patients and as very different from all other children. Support for parents may originate in their community where trusted connections have been made. Siblings benefit from understanding and assistance to thrive rather than trying to merely trying to survive. Integrating palliative care across all environments in which the child, parents, siblings, and others participate ensures that empathy and action replace the sympathy and despair that exist when good intentions do not have the opportunity to coincide with knowledge and tools to provide appropriate care. Effective communication between the child and family, health care providers, CHPCAs, school professionals, and other community organizations may ensure the best possible opportunity for the child and family to cope successfully.

Some of the apparent needs that may be addressed through a comprehensive, collaborative, CBPPC model include

- Effective pain and symptom management for the child that will support continued school participation. The school nurse may be equipped to better assess pain at school and provide prescribed medications when needed. After being taught nonpharmacologic interventions for pain and symptom control, scout leaders, youth pastors, and teachers can coach the child in deep breathing, progressive muscle relaxation, and guided imagery to afford an additional level of pain management and to engage the caring adult in direct support for the child.
- Anticipating the child's needs and establishing plans to address symptoms not yet present. The surgeon, PPC physician, or specialty nurse may provide information and education to empower school professionals, those at places of worship, Scout leaders, dance teachers, or chess club teachers with anticipatory guidance to help address concerns when the child undergoes an upcoming amputation.
- School social workers, counselors, faith leaders and others can help the ill child, siblings, and peers understand the diagnosis and that it is no one's fault that the child is sick.
- Specific strategies to reduce the child's anxiety about falling behind in school, such as posting assignments online, identifying a tutor to help the child when she or he returns to school, or setting up homebound education if the child must be gone longer.
- Unique ways to enable and enhance socialization with peers. Some children maintain social contacts despite a CCC; others have difficulty staying connected with friends and may privately grieve that loss. Each adult leader in the child's natural environments from school to worship to athletic teams to clubs has a responsibility to help the child transition in and out of that setting when the illness limits participation.
- Access and opportunities to participate in community or extracurricular activities. Caregivers in the child's natural environments often assume that the youngster is too sick to participate. With a collaborative CPPC model, including education and shared goal setting, the child's place in each environment is protected and the child is empowered to continue participation to the greatest extent possible.
- Opportunity for the child to live the life they want, to the greatest extent possible, as HCPs and others begin to understand the child's needs. Hope may be redefined to include a more significant school focus or the child may reconnect with his favorite sport by being the manager or statistician for the team.

Parent needs transcend all environments in which they, their ill child, and healthy siblings engage and can also be better met when HCPs and community partners collaborate:

- Parents often need support collaborating with specialists, understanding options for care, setting goals, and making decisions. A trusted spiritual leader may help parents and children in coping with the challenges imposed by a child's CCC or in bereavement support after a child's death.

- Parents and their children benefit considerably when teachers, coaches, spiritual leaders, piano teachers, Scout leaders, and a host of other adult caregivers take an interest in their healthy children. Providing extra care and support for the healthy siblings may afford parents a great deal of comfort and peace of mind in an otherwise chaotic situation.

Siblings usually share caregivers with the child who is ill and will also benefit when those individuals collaborate:

- Siblings will need help understanding the medical issues, communicating with their family, and learning to process and understand their emotions and concerns. Siblings are not often at the hospital when members of the palliative care team, who would usually provide that support (eg, social work, child life, music therapy), are present but do have access to the school counselor, music teacher, or the rabbi.
- Providing grief support around specific issues of loss. Children are not experienced in grieving and often hide their feelings. The natural environment provides trusted adults who may be best suited to support grieving siblings. In addition, when the sibling's grief is understood and managed in school, greater insight will exist regarding behaviors of the sibling when he or she is back in the classroom.

THE WHAT AND WHY OF THE COMPREHENSIVE PEDIATRIC PALLIATIVE CARE TEAM ACROSS ENVIRONMENTS

For all children, opportunities to grow, develop, and achieve are paramount to becoming a functional adult. Unlike most children, however, children with CCCs must work to try to be a normal child while existing in a very abnormal world for a child; a world that is focused on disease, death, fear, pain, and symptoms. The child must spend time away from home, family, preferred activities, and familiar, comforting people and places. In addition, this population of children may have concomitant behavioral, cognitive, or mobility challenges. Children in these circumstances need help.

The opportunity exists for professionals across all of the child's central environments, including school, athletics, theater, dance, Scouting, hospital, hospice, home health, and so on, to collaborate to provide optimal CPPC. The traditional medical model of PPC provides services in the hospital or in the child's home but does not address the child and family's need to obtain comprehensive support and care across other environments where they feel a familiarity and comfort with the people who are there. Although the people in the family's environment would like to help, they often do not know how to do so.

HCPs are encouraged to cast a wide net of collaboration to include educators, coaches, activity directors, faith leaders, and peers. With education and support in providing psychosocial palliative supports, those are the individuals who can begin to provide substantial care and support across all environments in which the child and family are involved. Ideally, a case manager would emerge from the local home health or CBPPC setting.

CBPPC, or care that is provided with the goal of offering PPC services in the community setting, is typically found in formal hospice or palliative care agencies or in home health programs.[28] CBPPC programs, when linked with hospital-based PPC programs, may be the optimal case management arm of CPPC. CBPPC is positioned to ensure comprehensive services, including continuity of care between hospital, outpatient PPC, and community-based services, including school, places of worship, and other activities. The CBPPC nurse or nurse clinician may be in a position that to provide strong case management for the child and family, and to act as a coordinator to merge services from a wide range of providers.

In the early stages of CPPC, the CBPPC nurse or other HCPs should provide information about palliation, developing goals of care, advance directives, and recommended accommodations at school, in sports, and other environments to the collaborative community partners. Soon, teachers, coaches, faith leaders, and others will share information with HCPs about the child in his or her natural environments, enabling HCPs to better understand the child and consider those issues most important to him or her when discussing treatment, goals of care, and advance care planning. An introductory face-to-face meeting of all adult leaders is requisite to the development of a collaborative CPPC team to truly integrate care across environments. After the initial meeting, updates and revisions can occur via email or phone.

Although the model of CPPC may already be practiced in some locations, there is no evidence that it has been studied or formalized. The time has come to begin the process of developing a formal, standards-based CPPC model of care. The first step is assessing the level of need among children and families, the willingness among community leaders and HCPs, and beginning the discussion of what a program may look like, who should be at the table, and next steps in development.

DO-NOT-ATTEMPT RESUSCITATION GOES TO SCHOOL

As in any new endeavor, there will be barriers and challenges to the development of an effective CPPC program. Addressing known barriers may serve to better prepare all stakeholders for possible hurdles. One known challenge to providing CPPC is out-of-hospital do-not-resuscitate (OOH DNAR) orders. Parents and children may request that their OOH DNAR order be honored at school, places of worship, and at the child's preferred activities. The OOH DNAR order emerges when the child, parents, and physicians decide to forego cardiopulmonary resuscitation (CPR) in the event the child's heart stops. It is extremely uncommon for community partners to be asked to honor an OOH DNAR order because it is rare for a school-aged child to confront the known possibility of failure of CPR. Most school districts are required to provide CPR until the emergency medical team (EMT) arrives and takes over, thus creating an especially challenging situation for school districts when a student and his family decide to exercise the child's right to refuse resuscitation.[29] Schools who previously were agreeable to PPC at school may now take a step backwards as they try to determine their liability and how to act in the child's best interest.

Good education to school staff, regarding all aspects of an OOH DNAR order, is critical. When it is invoked, the decision may be to continue other forms of medical therapies or to focus only on comfort care. It is important to note, however, that an OOH DNAR order addresses only resuscitation status and does not define all other goals of care.[30] Some children are too frail to come to school but others may choose to attend school as long as possible, especially when school has been a favored activity.

In 1994, the AAP issued guidelines on foregoing life-sustaining medical treatment, including CPR, for children and adolescents. The guidelines stated it is ethically acceptable to forego CPR when it is unlikely to be effective or when the risks outweigh the benefits, including the parents' and child's assessment of the child's quality of life.[31] More children with CCCs are going to school despite the barriers and challenges imposed by their diagnoses. Children and adolescents with life-limiting conditions may want to be with peers doing the things they enjoy.[32] Both IDEA and Section

504 provide federal legislation that guarantees that children with health care needs will be accommodated in school. Schools that are not in compliance face hefty monetary fines and other sanctions.

IDEA exempts schools from providing medical services but states that a child cannot be excluded from school on the grounds of needing intermittent care to participate.[32] It is important for parents, the student, and HCPs to request inclusion of services that address health issues within the individualized health care plan (IHCP). An IHCP can also be developed for children with 504 Plans, or even those with no plan, and may also include an emergency care plan. IHCPs represent an important safeguard for providing the health care needed by the student in the school environment. The IHCP is also protected by federal law because it is part of the student's educational individualized education program or 504 plan. The essential role of the licensed school nurse in the development and implementation of a student's IHCP is supported by the AAP.[32] The student's participation in school and extracurricular activities, and even their ability to be at school, is also supported by the IHCP.[33] Although schools are mandated to provide supplementary aids and health care services to accommodate the children, it is not the fault of schools that they cannot actually accomplish that in all circumstances.

Twenty years ago, it was rare for a school to honor a child's OOH DNAR order. Although more schools will honor the order on an individual basis today, there still are not many districts that have adopted policies or procedures. In 2005, an investigation reported that 80% of the nation's 50 largest school districts and districts in 31 additional state capitals did not have a policy, regulation, or protocol supporting a student's OOH DNAR order.[34] The application of an order at school may exceed the school's scope of decision-making. The school and specific staff members may risk liability if they choose to adhere to the order and not perform CPR. Without overarching local or state regulatory or legal framework the school may decide that it is bound to provide CPR.[34]

The arguments from schools regarding OOH DNAR orders have multiple tentacles. It has been argued that schools are not medical facilities. Teachers are lay persons, without medical training, being asked to determine if a cardiac or respiratory arrest is due to the underlying illness for which there is an order or if the child choked on a piece of meat at lunch. Educators express discomfort in trying to identify when and if the DNAR should be honored. Many educators have been trained in CPR and an OOH DNAR order imposes a directive that requires them to forego using their training in a situation in which they feel uncertainty. Others voice an unwillingness to stand around and do nothing for legal or personal moral reasons. An understanding of what palliative care is, and that it does not include doing nothing may aid in reformulating a concept of palliative care. Finally, another argument is that an arrest is a startling and frightening occurrence to observe and such an experience could be traumatic for observers and especially so for classmates. The counterargument is that unsuccessful CPR may also be traumatic.[35]

It is important that HCPs and the PPC team hear and acknowledge the concerns of school professionals and work to develop a plan that absolves school professionals from being decision-makers in an OOH DNAR order situation. The IHCP should clearly outline an action plan in case the event occurs at school. For example, the teacher can be in charge of getting the other children back to the classroom or staying with them in that location and providing them comfort. The administrator assists the school nurse in getting the child into the nurse's office and onto a cot. EMTs and parents are called by the school secretary. Other staff members may also be assigned roles. There may be opportunities for others to hold the child, provide supplemental oxygen, provide a blanket, or hold the child's hand. The school nurse and EMTs should be in control of direct patient care, if warranted.

SUMMARY

Despite the existence of a CCC, children remain dynamic beings who move through developmental stages of growth and continue to address the challenges of childhood as they work toward the goal of becoming an adult. Children with CCCs and their families require extensive support to achieve the best possible quality of life despite the child's serious health condition.

PPC has emerged over the past generation as an interdisciplinary model of health care that recognizes the unique challenges of children with CCCs. PPC is a service that only exists in a hospital or CBPPC agency even though children spend most of their time at home and in their communities of school, worship, play, activities, and sports.

A review of the current status of the needs of children with CCCs and their families identifies the opportunity to redefine palliative care beyond a medical model and to include the community environments where children spend most of their time. This includes partnering with caregivers in schools, places of worship, athletics, scouting, and other community activities.

A first step to providing CPPC services, across disciplines, is agreeing on a common language. A recommendation is to use the term CCC to describe children who benefit from PPC provided across disciplines. To distinguish this new type of palliative care for children from the purely medical model of PPC, the term CPPC is suggested for use when referring to the broad base of services for children provided across disciplines in the child's natural environment.

REFERENCES

1. Clinical Practice Guidelines for Quality Palliative Care, Third Edition. National Consensus Project for Quality Palliative Care; 2013. National Consensus Project for Quality Palliative Care. 2009. Available at: www.nationalconsensusproject.org/guidelines_download2.aspx. Accessed March 6, 2016.
2. NHPCO's Facts and Figures: Pediatric Palliative & Hospice Care in America. National Hospice and Palliative Care Organization. By Friebert S, Williams C. 2014. Available at: http://www.nhpco.org/sites/default/files/public/quality/Pediatric_Facts-Figures.pdf. Accessed February 20, 2016.
3. Palliative Care for Children. American Academy of Pediatrics. Committee on Bioethics and Committee on Hospital Care. Pediatrics 2000;106(2 Pt 1):351-7. Available at: http://pediatrics.aappublications.org/content/pediatrics/106/2/351.full.pdf.
4. Field MJ, Behrman RE, editors. When children die: improving palliative and end-of-life care for children and their families. Institute of Medicine of the National Academies. Washington, DC: The National Academies Press; 2003.
5. Dodge JA, Lewis PA, Stanton M, et al. Cystic fibrosis mortality and survival in the United Kingdom: 1947-2003. Eur Respir J 2007;29(3):522-6.
6. Wong LY, Paulozzi LJ. Survival of infants with spina bifida: a populations study; 1970-1994. Paediatr Perinat Epidemiol 2001;15(4):374-8.
7. Wise PH. The transformation of child health in the United States: Social disparities in child health persist despite dramatic improvements in child health overall. Health Aff (Millwood) 2004;23(5):9-25.

8. Eagle M, Baudouin SV, Chandler C, et al. Survival in Duchenne muscular dystrophy: improvements in life expectancy since 1967 and the impact of home nocturnal ventilation. Neuromuscul Disord 2002;12(10):926–9.

9. Lorenz J. Survival of the extremely preterm infant in North America in the 1990s. Clin Perinatol 2000;27(2):255–62.

10. Feudtner C, Hays R, Haynes G, et al. Deaths attributed to pediatric complex chronic conditions: National trends and implications for supportive care services. Pediatrics 2001;107(6):e99. Available at: http://pediatrics.aappublications.org/content/pediatrics/107/6/e99.full.pdf.

11. Feudtner C, Feinstein JA, Zhong W, et al. Pediatric complex chronic conditions classification system version 2: updated for ICD-10 and complex medical technology dependence and transplantation. BMC Pediatr 2014;14:199.

12. WHO Definition of Palliative Care: WHO Definition of Palliative Care for Children. World Health Organization Web site. 2016. Available at: http://www.who.int/cancer/palliative/definition/en/. Accessed March 19, 2016.

13. Section on Hospice and Palliative Medicine. What is Palliative Care? American Academy of Pediatrics Web site. Available at: https://www2.aap.org/sections/palliative/WhatIsPalliativeCare.html. Accessed February 13, 2016.

14. Standards of Practice for Pediatric Palliative Care and Hospice. National Hospice and Palliative Care Organization. Adapted from: Palliative Care for Children Pediatric Palliative Care by Morrow A. 2009. Available at: http://www.nhpco.org/sites/default/files/public/quality/Ped_Pall_Care%20_Standard.pdf.pdf. Accessed March 09, 2016.

15. Adolescents and Young Adults with Cancer. National Cancer Institute Web site. 2015. Available at: http://www.cancer.gov/types/aya. Accessed January 16, 2016.

16. Wolfe J, Klar N, Grier HE, et al. Understanding of prognosis among parents of children who died of cancer: impact on treatment goals and integration of palliative care. JAMA 2000;284(19):2469–75.

17. Mack JW, Joffe S. Communicating about prognosis: ethical responsibilities of pediatricians and parents. Pediatrics 2014;44(1):33–5.

18. Pediatric Palliative Care Referral Criteria. Center to Advance Palliative Care CAPC Web site. Prepared by Friebert S, Osenga K. 2009. Available at: https://central.capc.org/eco_download.php?id=588. Accessed February 6, 2016.

19. Feudtner C, Christakis DA, Connell FA. Pediatric deaths attributable to complex chronic conditions: a population-based study of Washington State, 1980-1997. Pediatrics 2000;106:205–9.

20. ChiPPS White Paper: A call for change: recommendations to improve the care of children living with life-threatening conditions. National Hospice and Palliative Care Organization. 2001. Available at: www.nhpco.org/sites/default/files/public/.../Pediatric_Facts-Figures.pdf. Accessed February 20, 2016.

21. McPherson M, Arango P, Fox H, et al. A new definition of children with special health care needs. Pediatrics 1998;102:137–40.

22. Grossman, LK & Duryea TK. Children with special health care needs. UpToDate. Topic 2840 Version 27.0. 2016. Available at: http://www.uptodate.com/contents/children-with-special-health-care-needs. Accessed May 22, 2016.

23. The National Survey of Children with Special Health Care Needs Chartbook 2009–2010. U.S. Department of Health and Human Services, Health Resources and Services Administration, Maternal and Child Health Bureau. Rockville (MD): U.S. Department of Health and Human Services; 2013.

24. Martin EW, Martin R, Terman DL. The legislative and litigation history of special education. Future Child 1996;6(1):25–39.
25. Thirty-five Years of Progress in Educating Children with Disabilities Through IDEA. U.S. Department of Education. Office of Special Education and Rehabilitative Services. 2010. Available at: http://www2.ed.gov/about/offices/list/osers/idea35/history/index_pg10.html. Accessed January 20, 2016.
26. Building the Legacy: IDEA 2004. Q and A: Questions and Answers on Individualized Education Programs (IEP's), Evaluations and Reevaluations ED.gov U.S. Department of Education. Available at: http://idea.ed.gov/. Accessed January 13, 2016.
27. Protecting Students with Disabilities. U.S. Department of Education. Office for Civil Rights. 2015. Available at: http://www2.ed.gov/about/offices/list/ocr/504faq.html. Accessed January 24, 2016.
28. Kaye EC, Rubenstein J, Levine D, et al. Pediatric palliative care in the community. CA Cancer J Clin 2015;65(4):316–33.
29. Adelman J. The school-based do-not-resuscitate order. DePaul J Health Care Law 2010;13(2):197–214.
30. Sanderson A, Zurakowski D, Wolfe J. Clinician perspectives regarding the do-not-resuscitate order. JAMA Pediatr 2013;167(10):954–8.
31. Guidelines on foregoing life-sustaining medical treatment. American Academy of Pediatrics, Committee on Bioethics. Pediatrics 1994;93(3):532–6.
32. Council on School Health and Committee on Bioethics, Murray RD, Antommaria AH. Honoring do-not-attempt-resuscitation requests in schools. Pediatrics 2010;125(5):1073–7.
33. Special education, School Health: Policy and Practice. 6th edition. Elk Grove Village, IL: American Academy of Pediatrics Committee on School Health; 2004. p. 51–75.
34. Kimberly MB, Forte AL, Carroll JM, et al. Pediatric do-not-attempt-resuscitation orders and public schools: a national assessment of policies and laws. Am J Bioeth 2005;5(1):59–65.
35. Compton S, Grace H, Madgy A, et al. Post-traumatic stress disorder symptomology associated with witnessing unsuccessful out-of-hospital cardiopulmonary resuscitation. Acad Emerg Med 2009;16(3):226–9.

A Review of Pediatric Telemental Health

Eve-Lynn Nelson, PhD[a,b,*], Susan Sharp, DO[c]

KEYWORDS

- Telemedicine • Telemental health • Behavioral health

KEY POINTS

- Because of the widening gap between need for child mental health services and availability of child specialists, secure videoconferencing options are more needed than ever.
- Based on a comprehensive review of real-time videoconferencing evidence to date, videoconferencing is an effective approach to improving access to behavioral health interventions for children and adolescents.
- Overall, telemental health is feasible and well accepted by families, and shows promise for disseminating evidence-based treatments to underserved communities.

INTRODUCTION

Because of chronic and worsening specialist shortages across pediatrics specialties as well as limited access to empirically supported interventions, telemedicine is becoming more widely adopted with children and adolescents, with telemental health among the most active pediatric specialties.[1–3] Telemedicine is defined as "the use of medical information exchanged from one site to another via electronic communications to improve patients' health status."[4] Telemental health, also called telebehavioral health, is an umbrella term to refer to all of the names and types of behavioral and mental health services that are provided via synchronous telecommunications technologies.[5,6] About 20% of US children and adolescents aged 9 to 17 years have diagnosable psychiatric disorders.[7] In addition, approximately 31% of children are affected by chronic conditions.[8] Many other youth show subthreshold symptoms and stress and grief reactions that benefit from intervention. Younger children are at risk for developmental and behavioral disorders. However, there are a growing number of evidence-based psychotherapy approaches to support children and their

Disclosures: None.
[a] KU Pediatrics, University of Kansas Medical Center, Kansas City, KS, USA; [b] University of Kansas Center for Telemedicine & Telehealth, 4330 Shawnee Mission Parkway, Suite 136, MS 7001, Fairway, KS 66205, USA; [c] Psychiatry & Behavioral Sciences Department, University of Kansas Medical Center, MS 4015, 3901 Rainbow Blvd, Kansas City, KS 66160, USA
* Corresponding author.
E-mail address: enelson2@kumc.edu

families in coping with the range of psychiatric presentations,[9–11] as well as pediatric psychology approaches for supporting children with acute and chronic medical conditions and their families.[12]

However, the supply of child behavioral health specialists trained in the latest clinical advances is very small, with demand far outpacing supply across child and adolescent psychiatrists,[13–15] child and adolescent therapists and other specialists,[16–19] and developmental medicine. Thus, most children with behavioral health concerns do not receive any therapy, let alone evidence-based treatments delivered by behavioral health specialists.[20] The rationale for telemental health is to bridge the gap between supply and demand, particularly in rural and other underserved communities that face declining economies, poor access to mental health insurance, and limited transportation options.[21,22] Telemental health helps increase regular attendance by diminishing the financial and temporal barriers of travel and time from work as well as offering access to therapists outside the community via health clinics and schools, which may be less stigmatizing than traditional mental health settings.

Telemental health services build on a long history of moving mental health care for youth from the mental health clinic to the community in order to increase access to care; decrease stigma; increase adherence to treatment planning; and, it is hoped, enhance effectiveness and care coordination in naturalistic settings. These community settings provide advantages in gathering information from multiple informants/supporters about the broad range of contextual factors influencing children's behaviors and mental health needs. In particular, telemental health offers a powerful opportunity for collaboration with pediatricians to help them address the increasing expectations to improve their skills in diagnosing and managing pediatric behavioral conditions.[3,23]

Although telemental health services initially focused on rural settings,[24] they are increasingly offered in diverse settings, including underserved parts of urban communities.[25] Mental health centers and other child-serving facilities may provide infrastructure that facilitates the implementation of telemental health services. Many schools are seeking to understand their students' mental health needs and are willing to use their videoconferencing systems to access telemental health services.[26] Most behavioral health diagnoses across the developmental spectrum have been evaluated through videoconferencing consistent with patients in usual outpatient practice.[5] Telemental health allows youth to be evaluated in their own communities accompanied by family or community members who may provide context and perspective that is not available if services are provided in distant health centers.[27] Primary care practices are often key partners in telemental health services.[3]

This article first summarizes the pediatric research to date across telemental health specialties.[5,28] Underscoring ethical considerations, it then presents a case study emphasizing ethical considerations in best practice.

SUMMARY OF TELEMENTAL HEALTH EVIDENCE WITH CHILDREN AND ADOLESCENTS

Studies were included if they (1) consisted of videoconferencing applications across the pediatric age range; (2) included psychiatry/pharmacotherapy, psychotherapy and/or a pediatric psychology intervention, and/or developmental medicine intervention; and (3) included videoconferencing as the method of intervention across assessment or treatment. Studies were excluded if they (1) were conducted using telephone or mobile interactions without video, (2) used Web-based or e-health interventions as a primary method for service delivery (ie, predominantly asynchronous Web-delivered content), and/or (3) focused solely on education/training or population description. These criteria were established in a previous review.[29] As presented in **Table 1**, the

Table 1
Telemental health intervention using videoconferencing

Study	Population	Sample Description and Sample Size	Study Design	Summary of Findings
Child Psychiatry Intervention Using Videoconferencing				
Elford et al,[30] 2000	Various diagnoses	n = 25 youth Age: 4–16 y	RCT, VC vs F2F	96% concordance between VC and F2F diagnostic evaluations, no difference in patient or parent satisfaction between VC and F2F, 91% of parents reported preference for VC to long-distance travel
Elford et al,[31] 2001	Various diagnoses	n = 23 youth	Descriptive, VC	Diagnosis and treatment recommendation were equal to usual, in-person care
Greenberg et al,[32] 2006	Various diagnoses	No children, 35 PCPs, 12 caregivers	Descriptive, focus groups with PCPs and caregivers	PCP and caregivers satisfied with VC and frustrated with limitations of local supports. Family caretakers and service providers frustrated with limitations of VC
Lau et al,[33] 2011	Various diagnoses	n = 45 youth Age: 3–17 y	Descriptive, VC	Use of VC showed a large variation in patient characteristics, such as age, current living situation, and psychological symptoms. The most common reason for VC referral was for diagnostic clarification (67%). Telepsychiatrists recommended a change in medication for most (80.8%) who were already on medication and to begin medications for those not on medication at time of consult (63.2%)
Myers et al,[34] 2006	Incarcerated adolescents	n = 115 youth Age: 14–18 y	Descriptive, VC satisfaction	80% successfully prescribed medications and expressed confidence in the psychiatrist by video, and youth expressed concerns about privacy
Myers et al,[35] 2007	Various diagnoses	n = 172 patients Age: 2–21 y 387 clinic visits	Descriptive, VC satisfaction	High satisfaction with services, more so with pediatricians vs family physicians
Myers et al,[36] 2010	Various diagnoses	n = 701 patients referred by 190 PCPs	Descriptive, use of VC	Pediatricians referred to VC services more frequently than family providers, reported VC as feasible, acceptable, and increasing access to mental health services

(continued on next page)

Table 1
(continued)

Study	Population	Sample Description and Sample Size	Study Design	Summary of Findings
Myers et al,[37] 2013	ADHD	n = 223 youths Age: 5.5–12.9 y	RCT, feasibility of VC	Demonstrated feasibility of conducting RCT with the use of VC with children living in underserved communities, clinicians showed high fidelity to treatment protocols, minor technical difficulties did not interfere with providing care
Myers et al,[38] 2015	ADHD, ODD, anxiety	n = 223 youth	RCT, VC vs F2F	Caregivers reported significantly greater improvement for inattention, hyperactivity, combined ADHD, ODD, and role performance for VC compared with those treated in primary care, teachers also reported significantly greater improvement in ODD and for performance for VC
Pakyurek et al,[39] 2010	Various diagnoses	n = 12 youth	Descriptive, VC vs F2F	VC may be superior to F2F for routine clinical consultation in primary care
Rockhill et al,[40] 2013	ADHD, ODD, anxiety	n = 223 children Telepsychiatrists and PCPs of these children	RCT	Telepsychiatrists adhered to guideline-based care, used higher medication doses than PCPs, and their patients reached target of 50% reduction in ADHD symptoms more often than with PCPs
Szeftel et al,[41] 2012	Developmental disability	n = 45 youth	Descriptive	VC led to changed psychiatric diagnosis for 70%; changed medication in 82% of patients initially, 41% at 1 y, and 46% at 3 y; VC helped PCPs with recommendations for developmental disabilities
Yellowlees,[42] 2008	Various diagnoses	n = 41 youth	VC pre-post	At 3 mo following psychiatric diagnostic evaluation, improvements in the Affect and Oppositional domains of the Child Behavior Checklist were observed
Myers et al,[43] 2004	Various diagnoses	n = 159 youth Age: 3–18 y	Comparison of patients evaluated using VC vs F2F	Demographically, clinically, and by reimbursement, patients look similar between VC and F2F, VC had greater adverse case mix

Study	Diagnosis/Population	Sample	Design	Findings
Myers et al,[44] 2008	Various diagnoses	n = parents of 172 youths	Descriptive, VC satisfaction	Satisfaction was higher in parents of school-aged children vs those with adolescents, high adherence for return appointments
Child Clinical Psychology Intervention Using Videoconferencing				
Fox et al,[45] 2008	Juvenile offenders	n = 190 youth Age: 12–19 y	VC pre-post	Youth increased goal achievement in areas of health, family, and social skills
Heitzman Powell et al,[46] 2014	Autism	n = 7 parents Youth age not reported	VC pre-post	Parents increased their knowledge and self-reported implementation of behavioral strategies
Himle et al,[47] 2012	Tic disorders	n = 18 youth Age: 8–17 y	RCT, VC vs F2F	Across groups, significant improvements in tic behaviors and strong ratings for acceptability and therapist/client alliance. No differences between treatment groups
Tse et al,[48] 2015	ADHD	n = 37 youth M (Teletherapy) = 9.15 y M (F2F) = 9.39 y	Substudy of larger clinical trial, VC vs F2F	Families in the 2 caregiver training conditions showed comparable attendance at sessions and satisfaction with their care. Caregivers in both conditions reported comparable outcomes for their children's ADHD-related behaviors and functioning, but caregivers in the teletherapy group did not report improvement in their own distress
Nelson et al,[49] 2006	Depression	n = 28 youth M = 10.3 y	RCT, VC vs F2F	Treatment yielded significant improvement for depression in both conditions, with no between-group differences
Nelson et al,[50] 2012	ADHD	n = 22 youth M = 9.3 y	VC feasibility	No factor inherent to the VC delivery mechanism impeded adherence to national ADHD guidelines
Reese et al,[51] 2012	ADHD	n = 8 youth M = 7.6 y	VC pre-post	Using group Triple P Positive Parenting Program instead of VC, families reported improved child behavior and decreased parent distress
Reese et al,[52] 2013	Autism	n = 21 youth	RCT, VC vs F2F	No difference in reliability of diagnostic accuracy, ADOS observations, ratings for ADI-R parent report or symptoms, and parent satisfaction

(continued on next page)

Table 1
(continued)

Study	Population	Sample Description and Sample Size	Study Design	Summary of Findings
Reese et al,[53] 2015	Autism	Autism Diagnostic Teams	VC feasibility	Using VC provided families in rural and underserved areas improved access to diagnostic services, parents equally satisfied with services received through VC and through university-based medical team
Stain et al,[54] 2011	Psychosis	n = 11 youth Age: 14–30 y	VC feasibility	Differences between VC and F2F modes of neuropsychological assessment were close to zero, VC produced higher ratings for general cognitive functioning (WTAR) compared with F2F assessments, strong acceptability of VC assessment from participants
Storch et al,[55] 2011	OCD	n = 31 youth Age: 7-16 y M = 11.1 y	Waitlist control, VC vs F2F	VC was superior to F2F on all primary outcome measures, with a significantly higher percentage of individuals in the VC group meeting remission criteria than in the F2F group
Xie et al,[56] 2013	ADHD	n = 22 parents Child M = 10.4 y	RCT, VC vs F2F	Parent training via VC showed same degree of improvement in disciplinary practices, ADHD symptoms, and overall functioning as F2F
Pediatric Psychology Intervention Using Videoconferencing				
Bensink et al,[57] 2008	Pediatric cancer	n = 8 youth Not reported	VC feasibility	Using VC rather than videophone to families with children diagnosed with cancer, the study noted technical feasibility and high parental satisfaction
Clawson et al,[58] 2008	Pediatric feeding disorders	n = 15 youth Age: 8 mo to 10 y old	VC feasibility	VC was feasible with the pediatric feeding disorder population and resulted in cost savings
Davis et al,[59] 2013	Pediatric obesity	n = 58 youth Age: 5–11 y M = 8.6 y	RCT, VC vs F2F physician visits	Both groups showed improvements in BMIz, nutrition, and physical activity, and the groups did not differ significantly on primary outcomes
Davis et al,[60] 2016	Pediatric obesity	n = 103 youth	RCT, VC vs telephone	Participants highly satisfied with both intervention methods, completion rates higher compared with other pediatric obesity interventions, both methods highly feasible

Study	Condition	Sample	Design	Findings
Freeman et al,[61] 2013	Diabetes adherence	n = 71 youth; VC M = 15.2 y; F2F M = 14.9 y	RCT, VC vs F2F	No differences in therapeutic alliance between the groups
Glueckauf et al,[62] 2002	Pediatric epilepsy	n = 22 (Youth); M = 15.4 y	RCT, VC, F2F, and telephone	All groups improved in psychosocial problem severity and frequency and child prosocial behavior, with no significant differences across groups. No differences in adherence between the groups were noted
Hommel et al,[63] 2013	IBD, adherence	n = 9 youth; M = 13.7 y	VC pre-post	The VC approach resulted in improved adherence and cost savings across patients
Lipana et al,[64] 2013	Pediatric obesity	n = 243 youth; M = 11 y	Pre-post, VC, and F2F	Using a nonrandomized design, the VC group showed more improvement than the F2F group in enhancing nutrition, increasing activity, and decreasing screen time
Morgan et al,[65] 2008	Congenital heart disease	n = 27 parents; Child age: 0–25 mo	RCT, VC, and telephone	The VC approach decreased parent anxiety significantly more than phone, and resulted in significantly greater clinical information
Mulgrew et al,[66] 2011	Pediatric obesity	n = 25 youth; Age: 4–11 y	VC feasibility	No significant difference in parent satisfaction between consultations for weight management delivered by VC or F2F
Shaikh et al,[67] 2008	Pediatric obesity	n = 99 youth; Age: 1–17 y	VC pre-post	VC consultations resulted in substantial changes/additions to diagnoses. For a subset of patients, repeated VC consultations led to improved health behaviors, weight maintenance, and/or weight loss
Wilkinson et al,[68] 2008	Cystic fibrosis	n = 16 youth; Not reported	RCT, videophone vs F2F	No significant differences in quality of life, anxiety levels, depression levels, admissions to hospital or clinic attendances, general practitioner calls, or intravenous antibiotic use between the 2 groups
Witmans et al,[69] 2008	Sleep disorders	n = 89; Age: 1–18 y	VC feasibility	Patients were very satisfied with the delivery of multidisciplinary pediatric sleep medicine services rather than VC

Abbreviations: ADHD, attention-deficit/hyperactivity disorder; ADI-R, Autism Diagnostic Interview, Revised; ADOS, Autism Diagnostic Observation Schedule; F2F, face to face; IBD, inflammatory bowel disorder; M, mean; OCD, Obsessive Compulsive Disorder; ODD, oppositional defiant disorder; PCPs, primary care providers; RCT, randomized controlled trial; VC, videoconferencing; WTAR, Wechsler Test of Adult Reading.

telemental health evidence is presented in 3 sections: child psychiatry, child clinical psychology, and pediatric psychology.

Child Psychiatry Intervention Using Videoconferencing

The literature specifically addressing telepharmacotherapy with children and adolescents is still emerging (see **Table 1**). Two retrospective chart reviews describe the results of telepsychiatry consultation. One study reviewed the charts of 223 patients and found that consultation resulted in changes in diagnosis (48%), treatment (81.6%), and clinical improvement (60.1%).[70] In the second study, 100 patient charts were reviewed after consultation. The results showed that consultation was associated with changes in diagnosis and treatment. Twenty-seven percent of those recommendations involved starting or managing medication. The medication classes included stimulants, antidepressants, and antipsychotics.[71]

There is only 1 pharmacologic treatment study reported.[38] Myers and colleagues[38] randomized 233 children diagnosed with attention-deficit/hyperactivity disorder (ADHD) to receive 22 weeks of treatment in one of 2 groups. The active control group received a single telepsychiatry consultation, with recommendations made to primary care providers (PCPs) to implement at their discretion during the trial. The intervention group received 6 sessions of pharmacotherapy via videoconferencing during the 22-week trial, complemented by caregiver behavior training delivered in person by a community therapist who was trained and supervised remotely. Findings suggest that the telepsychiatrists showed high fidelity to consensus-based pharmacotherapy algorithms. Participants in both the intervention and consultation groups improved, and those who received the 6-session intervention showed significantly better ADHD outcomes per caregivers' reports than did the consultation group. This study provides high-quality evidence for the ability to provide guideline-based care through videoconferencing and the added value that a short-term telepsychiatric intervention provides compared with a single teleconsultation to primary care. In addition, over the 8 weeks following participation in the trial, the treatment group had more follow-up sessions and active medication management by their PCPs, suggesting that a short-term intervention may also help PCPs improve their care for children with ADHD.

Child Clinical Interventions Using Videoconferencing

Table 1 summarizes the few studies that have addressed child clinical interventions using videoconferencing (see also Nelson and Patton,[72] 2016). Most studies are interventions for ADHD but also include a variety of single-study examples. Innovative research is emerging concerning home-based telemedicine for pediatric OCD.[73] Intervention approaches varied from focus on the youth to focus on the parent and ranged from feasibility trials to pre-post designs, and a handful of randomized controlled trials. Consistent with the more robust adult individual therapy literature, findings were overall positive related to feasibility, satisfaction, and outcome.[74,75] A recent study showed that the American Academy of Pediatrics' practice guidelines for the treatment of ADHD[76] can be reliably implemented in the school setting through videoconferencing.[50]

Pediatric Psychology Intervention Using Videoconferencing

As presented in **Table 1**, 13 studies spanned a wide range of chronic and acute childhood illnesses and used multiple pediatric psychology interventions, such as cognitive-behavioral strategies to promote coping and strategies to enhance treatment adherence. As with individual therapies, findings were overall positive for feasibility, satisfaction, and outcome, although definitive statements are difficult in light of the limited number of studies, small sample sizes, and limited replication.

Evidence Table Summary

Overall, there is a growing consensus that telemental health is a reasonable alternative to in-person behavioral health management of youth who do not have regular access to expert care.[72,77] It offers a new approach to collaborate with PCPs in meeting the increasing expectation that they manage common psychiatric disorders of childhood and adolescence in their practices[3,5] and intervene early. Some providers have suggested that telemental health may be especially suited for youth who are accustomed to the technology, especially adolescents who may respond to the personal space and feeling of control allowed by videoconferencing.[28,78] There is some preliminary evidence that videoconferencing offers advantages, including less self-consciousness, increased personal space, and decreased confidentiality concerns because the provider is outside the local community.[47]

BEST PRACTICES USING VIDEOCONFERENCING

Most individual therapy and pediatric psychology interventions using videoconferencing are intended to approximate the same high-quality services that are offered in the face-to-face setting. However, ethical considerations are magnified in the telemedicine setting because of its focus on reaching underserved and vulnerable populations. Thus, just as in on-site clinical settings, therapists must look to their professional ethics codes for guidance and the core ethical concern to protect the patient remains paramount.[6,79] Guidelines are emerging to inform reasonable steps for videoconferencing-based practice across clinical, administrative, and technical considerations. These guidelines include those from the American Academy of Child and Adolescent Psychiatry,[9] the American Psychological Association,[80] and the American Telemedicine Association.[5,78,81] Pediatrics guidelines are also helpful in informing child telemental health best practices and collaborative opportunities.[1]

Behavioral health providers are encouraged to seek ongoing training and mentorship to develop and maintain telemental health competencies, with careful consideration of clinical, technical, community engagement, and cultural competencies.[6,82] Resources are available both through the federally funded telehealth resource centers (www.telehealthresourcecenter.org) and other programs (eg, www.tmhguide.org, www.americantelemed.org). In order to maximize adherence and outcomes, the same attention to rapport and relationship building should be given in the telemental health setting as in the traditional clinic experience.[83] In addition, the telemental health service should carefully consider patient inclusion and exclusion criteria based on the needs of the referring clinicians, judgment of the teleprovider, and resources at the patient site, including the site's ability to attend to acutely suicidal or agitated patients.[5]

To better describe best practices, this article incorporates ethical approaches within the following case study that spans telemental health teams.

CASE EXAMPLE

The case example includes presentation, technology and setting, initial session, abbreviated history and case formulation, assessment, and treatments. Each telemedicine service seeing the patient and family is described: child psychiatry, child psychology, autism diagnostic clinic, and pediatric weight management.

Presentation

Jay is a 5-year-old boy referred to the telemental health specialists by his rural school, supported by his primary care physician. He presented to the rural special education center cooperative with his mother Karen and his stepfather Sean. Presenting concerns included oppositional behaviors at home and at school, symptoms of ADHD, and broader behavioral/developmental concerns based on the family history.

The family was given options for behavioral health services: to be seen through the local mental health center, although there were no child-trained psychiatrists or psychologists within their region; to see specialists in person at the academic health center; or to use videoconferencing. The telemental health option was appealing because of convenience and decreased family costs related to travel. In addition, the family had sought services through the community mental health center, which focused on individual play therapy with Jay; the family had not found this effective in addressing the presenting oppositional concerns. The availability of services at the hospital through telemental health was particularly appealing because it had less of the stigma or concern of being identified by other community members compared with visiting the mental health center. With his parent's consent, the teleproviders have collaborated with Jay's PCP across treatment.

The telemedicine nurse coordinator is the site champion at the special education cooperative, serving 15 different school districts. As such, she is competent in the telemedicine technology, the administrative expectations around confidentiality, and child behavioral health. She completed training around both the telemedicine and the mental health components of the clinic.[84] Before the appointment, she explained to Jay and his family what to expect in the telemental health visit and helped the family complete the paperwork, including consent to treatment, registration form, insurance information, Health Information Portability and Accountability Act–related Notice of Privacy, history intake form, behavioral questionnaires, records of medical care and prior medication trials, and laboratory values. The coordinator is available to assist the family throughout the telemental health encounters, particularly if there are any technical difficulties or emergent clinical concerns such as suicidal intent. She assists with supervising Jay outside the telemedicine room to allow his parents to talk with the teleproviders privately for part of the sessions.

Technology and Setting

Jay is seen over secure videoconferencing, connecting the child psychiatrist, child psychologist, developmental medicine team, and weight management team at the academic health center with the school in a small rural community. Coordination across patient/family, rural site, and provider schedules across different time zones is accomplished through the telemedicine office's scheduler. In this setting, standards-based videoconferencing systems were used on both sides using H.323 protocols. The hub/provider site uses a large room–based videoconferencing system using high-speed fiber connections and the spoke/rural site uses a room-based videoconferencing system over a cable modem, with connection speed limited by this lower bandwidth. Although technical difficulties have been minor and solved by rebooting the system, the provider and the rural sites benefited from having a readily accessible, consumer-focused technician to support sessions.

The teleprovider can zoom in on the patient to understand his speech and note motor functioning and affect. The quiet, private clinic space is large enough to accommodate both Jay and family members. A fax machine is close to the therapy room in order to exchange questionnaires, handouts, and therapy activities. The camera is placed strategically to see Jay seated at a small table in the room and the lighting allows the therapist to easily observe facial expressions.

Initial Sessions

Lessons are drawn from the initial sessions with both the child psychiatrist and child psychologist (or the teleproviders). Following well-established protocols tailored to each local site, the teleprovider socialized Jay and his guardian to the videoconferencing system, noting that it may take time to acclimate to the technology and not talk over each other. She informed the family that no one else could access the videoconferencing encounter and that the session was not being recorded. With the help of the site coordinator, the therapist explained how the components of the technology worked. The teleprovider reviewed informed consent components (ie, confidentiality and its limits around safety and abuse), risks and limitations associated with videoconferencing services, documentation procedures, and patient responsibilities around attendance and payment. As established ahead of time, the telephone was used as a backup in the rare event that the videoconferencing did not connect. Attention was given to rapport building, including Jay showing his recent drawing to the telemedicine team.

Abbreviated History

Karen described Jay as overall a smart, healthy, active boy. She reported a normal pregnancy and delivery. Developmental milestones were overall on time with the exception of speech/language. Jay had multiple ear infections with tubes placed and adenoids removed at age 2 years. Additional medical history was unremarkable with the exception of a febrile seizure at 3 years old. He has seasonal allergies and asthma, with medications including steroids and albuterol.

Jay receives speech and language services through his Individualized Education Plan. No concerns were noted with gross or fine motor skills. He has difficulty playing with other children because, if he does not get his way, he screams at other children or falls down on the ground. He is advanced in general intelligence and academic skills. He has a short attention span and often does not follow simple instructions. Karen described that Jay shows ADHD symptoms, including difficulty sitting still, fidgetiness, impulsiveness, forgetfulness, and disorganization. He has low frustration tolerance and has daily outbursts at home and school in which he swings his arms and yell. He does not destroy property and does not become aggressive. Tantrums last from a few minutes up to hours.

He argues with his teacher and other school personnel constantly, and is difficult to redirect. Jay readily answered questions over the videoconferencing system and describes himself as happy overall despite having few friends. He blames others for things he does and often lies. He is described as moody, but does not make negative self-comments or show suicidal ideation/planning. He is described as eating constantly and his body mass index places him as overweight. He has difficulty transitioning at bedtime but little trouble falling or staying asleep once in bed.

Jay had no contributing past medical or psychiatric history. No concerns were noted in relation to anxiety, psychosis, or mania. With regard to possible autism spectrum disorder, there is history of language delay, but he is noted to have empathy, social reciprocity, and no restricted interests or repetitive behaviors. He resides with his parents and 2-year-old brother. Family history was positive for ADHD and Asperger disorder in his maternal uncle. His mother had anxiety in the past, and depression on her side of the family.

Assessment and Case Formulation

Jay scored in the clinical range on the Vanderbilt Parent and Teacher Assessment Scales for ADHD and for oppositional defiant disorder (ODD),[85] which was also consistent with parent and school report

He also scored in these clinical ranges on the Swanson, Nolan and Pelham Teacher and Parent Rating Scale–Fourth Version (SNAP-IV) parent and teacher scales.[86] These results are similar to the narrative descriptions completed by his parents and teachers.

Interventions

The telemedicine treatment approaches across child psychiatry, child clinical psychology, autism assessment, and weight management are described here.

Child psychiatry

The child psychiatrist worked with the telemedicine coordinator to implement best practices around medication management, including tracking vital signs and weight, obtaining rating scales, checking metabolic laboratory work, and monitoring for adverse effects at each session.[87] After establishing the relationship, the telepsychiatrist effectively gathered all key elements of the psychiatric evaluation. On mental status, Jay was hyper and impulsive. He appeared distractible during the interview, but with bright affect and happy mood. There were no hallucinations or suicidal or homicidal ideations. Based on history, rating scales, and presentation, he was diagnosed with ADHD and ODD. After discussing risks, benefits, and potential side effects, he was prescribed Adderall XR 5 mg and his family agreed to a trial of this medicine. The family was given ways to reach his psychiatrist between appointments in case of need for interim care.

Educating his family has been an important part of treatment, including discussion of the diagnoses, prognosis, and treatment options. For example, the family was directed to CHADD.org and parentsmedguide.org as useful Web sites that address frequently asked questions and give resources to parents to help in the management of ADHD and other illnesses. Prescriptions for the schedule II medications were mailed to the patient's home. The child psychiatrist provided clear direction and her office contact number for interim needs such as requesting refills, asking questions, and reporting adverse effects.

At each follow-up appointment, it is helpful to have teacher and parent forms to quantify whether there is improvement. He was seen a month later and appeared to have improvement on the medicine, including improved ability to sit still and focus at school, and decreased number of outbursts. At 2-month follow-up, the parent reported that he had become more hyper and impulsive, and that outbursts had increased in frequency. The dose of Adderall XR was increased to 10 mg to better manage his symptoms. His parent called 3 months later to report that the increased dose again helped at first, but effects wear off over time. At the next appointment, Jay's medicine was switched to Concerta 18 mg and the family reported continued improvement at the follow-up, including better focus and decreased arguing. Jay will continue to follow in telemedicine as long as his family and clinician think it is helpful and practical. Once stabilized, some families elect to transition care back to their PCPs with consultation between the PCP and psychiatrist as needed.

Child clinical psychology

Treatment followed best practices for ADHD and ODD management.[88] Psychotherapy focused on evidence-based behavioral interventions, including sharing resources from *Parenting the Strong-Willed Child*[89] with the family. Initial discussion reinforced close supervision of Jay in order to catch him being good, redirect him quickly, and keep him on routine. The family increased special time with Jay and were encouraged to target key behaviors and "pick battles," with an emphasis on decreasing lecture/verbal attention for negative behaviors. Sessions included review/practice of time-out as well as use of a behavioral chart system to reinforce contingencies. Jay responded well to the sticker chart and worked to earn time on his iPad. A system of tracking behaviors and matching with rewards/consequences was established between home and school, with target behaviors including (1) making good choices with classmates (eg, no hitting, name calling), (2) following instructions, and (3) using an indoor voice (eg, no yelling). As in face-to-face settings, individual time with Jay focused on anger management strategies and social skills training. He was very engaged in role playing scenarios, more so than videoconferencing, particularly practicing steps on how to make friends and how to think through walking away when he is angry.

Autism diagnostic team

Because of Jay's family history of autism spectrum disorder and his poor social skills, his parents elected to have him tested through a special telemedicine program through his school. An innovative integrated services model is used to connect families and local school teams with the interdisciplinary team at the academic health center.[53] In the integrated model, trained autism diagnostic teams complete the autism measures on site at the school in order to examine characteristics of autism, including observation, play-based assessments, and parent interview. The local team then presents findings to the parents and developmental medicine team, who make the final diagnostic determination via telemedicine. Although Jay has some peer problems and behavioral rigidity and is reported to have some lack of empathy, Jay did not meet the criteria for autism spectrum disorder. The team reinforced the medication management and behavioral health strategies in order to control ADHD and oppositional behaviors.

Pediatric psychology

As Jay's initial behavioral health concerns have improved, his family expressed interest in additional supports related to managing his weight because he is in the overweight category. He completed an initial session via telemedicine with the Healthy Hawks team, including a psychologist, physician, and dietician. The focus is on holistic healthy lifestyle activities across the family.[60] The school team participation has helped integrate the healthy lifestyle approaches at home and school and reinforce healthy choices. In addition to one-on-one telemedicine visits, his family also plans to participate in an upcoming telemedicine group opportunity through Jay's school, which connects families at several schools to the intervention team at the academic health center.

Case Study Summary

The case study shows how telemental health services can reduce barriers to treatment. This case is noteworthy in the availability to see a specialist at a young age and the anticipated decreased in morbidity associated with poorly controlled behavioral health concerns. Although most elements of a visit are the same as in-person care, videoconferencing offers both unique advantages and challenges compared with in-person care. The teleproviders were able to ascertain adequate information at the initial visit to assist with a diagnosis and treatment plan. The patient and family quickly acclimated to the technology-supported environment and good rapport was established. From the teleproviders' perspectives, a major advantage of the videoconferencing system was the increased communication with a range of team participants, including extended family, primary care personnel, and school personnel, and the opportunity for input during assessment, treatment, and treatment maintenance. Adherence to regular follow-up visits was likely enhanced by the convenience of videoconferencing. However, creativity and planning ahead were required in order to share materials and to modify patient education strategies for videoconferencing.

Another advantage was health care trainee participation at the academic health center. A graduate psychology student assisted throughout the assessment and treatment and residents from both child psychiatry and pediatrics were able to observe a telemedicine session. The trainees had no prior exposure to working with rural populations or with telemedicine and it is hoped that the experience will increase interest in working with underserved families in the future.[90] In addition, the telemedicine site uses the videoconferencing setup not only to provide therapy services but also to support staff education around child behavioral health topics. Lunch-and-learn programs and other brief distance education offerings have helped the videoconferencing services grow quickly by helping personnel identify behavioral concerns and develop a positive professional relationship with the teleproviders.

SUMMARY

Because of the widening access gap to child behavioral health services, telemental health options are more needed than ever. Although the limited studies to date are encouraging, research is needed to better understand the unique advantages and disadvantages of services using videoconferencing. Research is especially needed in assessing adult models of care for children, including telemental health services in unsupervised settings such as the home.[91] Emerging guidelines inform ethical best practices in providing therapy using videoconferencing, with continued emphasis on care based on patient and parents' preferences, developmental and diagnostic considerations, personnel and other resources at the remote site, and therapist comfort.[44] As shown by the case example, telemental health has great potential to increase access to evidence-based assessment and treatment across behavioral health services for youth living in underserved communities.

New telemedicine approaches to meeting this demand are also needed, as well as meeting expectations for enhanced care coordination among primary care and behavioral health providers as part of medical home initiatives. The Patient Protection and Affordable Care Act has called for the meaningful use of telehealth technologies to improve health care and population health for all citizens.[92] Collaborative care models in which the behavioral health professional, most often a psychiatrist, and PCP jointly manage a population of patients with a care manager have been descried with adults,[93,94] and have potential for incorporation into the pediatric medical home.[2,95] In addition, telementoring models such as Project ECHO (Extension for Community Healthcare Outcomes) use telemedicine technology to support collaboration between specialist teams and PCPs in providing high-quality interventions for child behavioral health concerns.[96]

ACKNOWLEDGMENTS

The authors who like to acknowledge the valuable contribution of Ali Calkins, MA, research assistant at University of Kansas Center for Telemedicine & Telehealth in authoring this review.

REFERENCES

1. Burke BL, Hall RW. Telemedicine: pediatric applications. Pediatrics 2015;136(1): e293–308.
2. American Academy of Pediatrics. Committee on Pediatric Workforce. 2015. Available at: https://www.aap.org/en-us/about-the-aap/Committees-Councils-Sections/Pages/Committee-on-Pediatric-Workforce.aspx. Accessed May 1, 2016.

3. Goldstein F, Myers K. Telemental health: a new collaboration for pediatricians and child psychiatrists. Pediatr Ann 2014;43(2):79–84.
4. American Telemedicine Association (ATA) nomenclature. Available at: http://www.americantelemed.org/resources/nomenclature#T. Accessed May 1, 2016.
5. Cain S, Nelson E, Myers K. Telemental health. In: Dulcan MK, editor. Dulcan's textbook of child and adolescent psychiatry. Washington, DC: American Psychiatric Publishing; 2015. p. 1–18.
6. Luxton D, Nelson E, Maheu M. A Practitioner's guide to telemental health. Washington, DC: American Psychological Association Press; 2016.
7. Centers for Disease Control and Prevention (CDC). Mental health surveillance among children—United States, 2005–2011. MMWR Surveill Summ 2013;62:1–35.
8. Newacheck PW, Taylor WR. Childhood chronic illness: prevalence, severity, and impact. Am J Public Health 1992;82:364–71.
9. Myers KM, Cain S. Workgroup on quality. Practice parameter for telepsychiatry with children and adolescents. J Am Acad Child Adolesc Psychiatry 2008; 47(12):1468–83.
10. Dulcan MK. Dulcan's textbook of child and adolescent psychiatry. Washington, DC: American Psychiatric Publishing; 2015.
11. Weisz JR, Kazdin AE, editors. Evidence-based psychotherapies for children and adolescents. 2nd edition. New York: Guilford Press; 2010.
12. Roberts MC, Aylward BS, Wu YP, editors. Clinical practice of pediatric psychology. New York: Guilford; 2014.
13. Association of American Medical Colleges, Center for Workforce Studies. Physician specialty data book. Washington, DC: Association of American Medical Colleges; 2012. Available at: https://www.aamc.org/download/313228/data/2012physicianspecialtydatabook.pdf. Accessed May 1, 2016.
14. Flaum M. Telemental health as a solution to the widening gap between supply and demand for mental health services. In: Myers K, Turvey C, editors. Telemental health: clinical, technical and administrative foundations for evidence-based practice. London: Elsevier; 2013. p. 11–25.
15. Thomas CR, Holzer CE. The continuing shortage of child and adolescent psychiatrists. J Am Acad Child Adolesc Psychiatry 2006;45(9).1023–31.
16. American Psychological Association. APA survey of psychology health service providers. Washington, DC: American Psychological Association; 2008. Available at: http://www.apa.org/workforce/publications/08-hsp/index.aspx. Accessed May 1, 2016.
17. American Psychological Association. Underserved population: practice setting matters, 2011. Available at: http://www.apa.org/workforce/snapshots/2011/underserved-population.pdf. Accessed May 1, 2016.
18. Kazdin AE, Blase SL. Rebooting psychotherapy research and practice to reduce the burden of mental illness. Perspect Psychol Sci 2011;6(1):21–37.
19. Michalski DS, Kohout JL. The state of the psychology health service provider workforce. Am Psychol 2011;66(9):825–34.
20. Merikangas KR, He JP, Burstein M, et al. Service utilization for lifetime mental disorders in U.S. adolescents: results of the National Comorbidity Survey-Adolescent Supplement (NCS-A). J Am Acad Child Adolesc Psychiatry 2011;50:32–45.
21. Comer JS, Barlow DH. The occasional case against broad dissemination and implementation: retaining a role for specialty care in the delivery of psychological treatments. Am Psychol 2014;69:1–18.
22. Smalley B, Warren J, Rainer J, editors. Rural mental health. New York: Springer; 2012.

23. American Academy of Pediatrics. The new morbidity revisited: a renewed commitment to the psychosocial aspects of pediatric care. Pediatrics 2001; 108(5):1227–30.
24. Duncan AB, Velasquez SE, Nelson EL. Using videoconferencing to provide psychological services to rural children and adolescents: A review and case example. J Clin Child Adolesc Psychol 2014;43(1):115–27.
25. Spaulding R, Cain S, Sonnenschein K. Urban telepsychiatry: uncommon service for a common need. Child Adolesc Psychiatr Clin N Am 2011;20(1):29–39.
26. Stephan SH, Lever N, Bernstein L, et al. Telemental health in schools. J Child Adolesc Psychopharmacol 2016;26(3):266–72.
27. Savin D, Glueck DA, Chardavoyne J, et al. Bridging cultures: child psychiatry via videoconferencing. Child Adolesc Psychiatr Clin N Am 2011;20(1):125–34.
28. Nelson EL, Bui T. Rural telepsychology services for children and adolescents. J Clin Psychol 2010;66(5):490–501.
29. Van Allen J, Davis AM, Lassen S. The use of telemedicine in pediatric psychology: research review and current applications. Child Adolesc Psychiatr Clin N Am 2011;20:55–66.
30. Elford DR, White H, Bowering R, et al. A randomized controlled trial of child psychiatric assessments conducted using videoconferencing. J Telemed Telecare 2000;6:73–82.
31. Elford DR, White H, St. John K, et al. A prospective satisfaction study and cost analysis of a pilot child telepsychiatry service in Newfoundland. J Telemed Telecare 2001;7:73–81.
32. Greenberg N, Boydell KM, Volpe T. Pediatric telepsychiatry in Ontario: caregiver and service provider perspectives. J Behav Health Serv Res 2006;33(1):105–11.
33. Lau ME, Way BB, Fremont WP. Assessment of SUNY Upstate Medical University's child telepsychiatry consultation program. Int J Psychiatry Med 2011;42(1):93–104.
34. Myers K, Valentine J, Morganthaler R, et al. Telepsychiatry with incarcerated youth. J Adolesc Health 2006;38(6):643–8.
35. Myers K, Valentine JM, Melzer SM. Feasibility, acceptability, and sustainability of telepsychiatry for children and adolescents. Psychiatr Serv 2007;58:1493–6.
36. Myers KM, Vander Stoep A, McCarty CA, et al. Child and adolescent telepsychiatry: variations in utilization, referral patterns and practice trends. J Telemed Telecare 2010;16:128–33.
37. Myers K, Vander Stoep A, Lobdell C. Feasibility of conducting a randomized controlled trial of telemental health with children diagnosed with attention-deficit/hyperactivity disorder in underserved communities. J Child Adolesc Psychopharmacol 2013;23(6):372–8.
38. Myers K, Vander Stoep A, Zhou C, et al. Effectiveness of a telehealth service delivery model for treating attention-deficit/hyperactivity disorder: a community-based randomized controlled trial. J Am Acad Child Adolesc Psychiatry 2015; 54(4):263–74.
39. Pakyurek M, Yellowlees P, Hilty D. The child and adolescent telepsychiatry consultation: can it be a more effective clinical process for certain patients than conventional practice? Telemed J E Health 2010;16(3):289–92.
40. Rockhill C, Violette H, Vander Stoep A, et al. Caregivers' distress: Youth with attention-deficit/hyperactivity disorder and comorbid disorders assessed via telemental health. J Child Adolesc Psychopharmacol 2013;23(6):379–85.
41. Szeftel R, Federico C, Hakak R, et al. Improved access to mental health evaluation for patients with developmental disabilities using telepsychiatry. J Telemed Telecare 2012;18(6):317–21.

42. Yellowlees PM, Hilty DM, Marks SL, et al. A retrospective analysis of a child and adolescent eMental Health program. J Am Acad Child Adolesc Psychiatry 2008; 47(1):103–7.
43. Myers KM, Sulzbacher S, Melzer SM. Telepsychiatry with children and adolescents: are patients comparable to those evaluated in usual outpatient care? Telemed J E Health 2004;10:278–85.
44. Myers KM, Valentine JM, Melzer SM. Child and adolescent telepsychiatry: utilization and satisfaction. Telemed J E Health 2008;14(2):131–7.
45. Fox KC, Conner P, McCullers E, et al. Effect of a behavioural health and specialty care telemedicine programme on goal attainment for youths in juvenile detention. J Telemed Telecare 2008;14(5):227–30.
46. Heitzman-Powell LS, Buzhardt J, Rusinko LC, et al. Formative evaluation of an ABA outreach training program for parents of children with autism in remote areas. Focus Autism Other Dev Disabl 2013;29:23–38.
47. Himle MB, Freitag M, Walther M, et al. A randomized pilot trial comparing videoconference versus face-to-face delivery of behavior therapy for childhood tic disorders. Behav Res Ther 2012;50:565–70.
48. Tse YJ, McCarty CA, Vander Stoep A, et al. Teletherapy delivery of caregiver behavior training for children with attention-deficit hyperactivity disorder. Telemed J E Health 2015;21(6):451–8.
49. Nelson E, Barnard M, Cain S. Feasibility of teletherapy for childhood depression. Counsell Psychother Res 2006;6(3):191–5.
50. Nelson EL, Duncan A, Peacock G, et al. School-based telemedicine and adherence to national guidelines for ADHD evaluation. Psychol Serv 2012;9(3):293–7.
51. Reese RJ, Slone NC, Soares N, et al. Telehealth for underserved families: an evidence-based parenting program. Psychol Serv 2012;9(3):320–2.
52. Reese RM, Jamison R, Wendland M, et al. Evaluating interactive videoconferencing for assessing symptoms of autism. Telemed J E Health 2013;19(9):671–7.
53. Reese RM, Braun MJ, Hoffmeier S, et al. Preliminary evidence for the integrated systems using telemedicine. Telemed J E Health 2015;21(7):581–7.
54. Stain HJ, Payne K, Thienel R, et al. The feasibility of videoconferencing for neuropsychological assessments of rural youth experiencing early psychosis. J Telemed Telecare 2011;17(6):328–31.
55. Storch EA, Caporino NE, Morgan JR, et al. Preliminary investigation of web-camera delivered cognitive-behavioral therapy for youth with obsessive-compulsive disorder. Psychiatry Res 2011;189(3):407–12.
56. Xie Y, Dixon JF, Yee OM, et al. A study on the effectiveness of videoconferencing on teaching parent training skills to parents of children with ADHD. Telemed J E Health 2013;19(3):192–9.
57. Bensink M, Armfield N, Irving H, et al. A pilot study of videotelephone-based support for newly diagnosed paediatric oncology patients and their families. J Telemed Telecare 2008;14:315–21.
58. Clawson B, Selden M, Lacks M, et al. Complex pediatric feeding disorders: using teleconferencing technology to improve access to a treatment program. Pediatr Nurs 2008;34(3):213–6.
59. Davis AM, Sampilo M, Gallagher KS, et al. Treating rural pediatric obesity through telemedicine: outcomes from a small randomized controlled trial. J Pediatr Psychol 2013;38(9):932–43.
60. Davis AM, Sampilo M, Gallagher KC, et al. Treating rural pediatric obesity through telemedicine vs. telephone: outcomes from a cluster randomized controlled trial. J Telemed Telecare 2016;22(2):86–95.

61. Freeman KA, Duke DC, Harris MA. Behavioral health care for adolescents with poorly controlled diabetes via Skype: does working alliance remain intact? J Diabetes Sci Technol 2013;7(3):727–35.
62. Glueckauf RL, Fritz SP, Ecklund-Johnson EP, et al. Videoconferencing-based family counseling for rural teenagers with epilepsy: phase 1 findings. Rehabil Psychol 2002;47(1):49–72.
63. Hommel KA, Hente E, Herzer M, et al. Telehealth behavioral treatment for medication nonadherence: a pilot and feasibility study. Eur J Gastroenterol Hepatol 2013;25(4):469–73.
64. Lipana LS, Bindal D, Nettiksimmons J, et al. Telemedicine and face-to-face care for pediatric obesity. Telemed J E Health 2013;19(10):806–8.
65. Morgan RD, Patrick AR, Magaletta P. Does the use of telemental health alter the treatment experience? Inmates' perceptions of telemental health versus face-to-face treatment modalities. J Consult Clin Psychol 2008;76:158–62.
66. Mulgrew KW, Shaikh U, Nettiksimmons J. Comparison of parent satisfaction with care for childhood obesity delivered face-to-face and by telemedicine. Telemed J E Health 2011;17:383–7.
67. Shaikh U, Cole SL, Marcin JP, et al. Clinical management and patient outcomes among children and adolescents receiving telemedicine consultations for obesity. Telemed J E Health 2008;14(5):434–40.
68. Wilkinson OM, Duncan-Skingle F, Pryor JA, et al. A feasibility study of home telemedicine for patients with cystic fibrosis awaiting transplantation. J Telemed Telecare 2008;14(4):182–5.
69. Witmans MB, Dick B, Good J, et al. Delivery of pediatric sleep services via telehealth: the Alberta experience and lessons learned. Behav Sleep Med 2008;6:207–19.
70. Marcin JP, Nesbitt TS, Cole SL, et al. Changes in diagnosis, treatment, and clinical improvement among patients receiving telemedicine consultations. Telemed J E Health 2005;11(1):36–43.
71. Boydell KM, Volpe T, Kertes A, et al. A review of the outcomes of the recommendations made during paediatric telepsychiatry consultations. J Telemed Telecare 2007;13(6):277–81.
72. Nelson E, Patton S. Using videoconferencing to deliver individual therapy and pediatric psychology interventions with children and adolescents. J Child Adolesc Psychopharmacol 2016;26(3):212–20.
73. Comer JS, Furr JM, Cooper-Vince CE, et al. Internet-delivered, family-based treatment for early-onset OCD: a preliminary case series. J Clin Child Adolesc Psychol 2014;43(1):74–87.
74. Gros DF, Morland LA, Greene CJ, et al. Delivery of evidence-based psychotherapy via video telehealth. J Psychopathol Behav Assess 2013;35(4):506–21.
75. Hilty DM, Ferrer DC, Parish MB, et al. The effectiveness of telemental health: a 2013 review. Telemed J E Health 2013;19:444–54.
76. American Academy of Pediatrics. Clinical practice guideline: diagnosis and evaluation of the child with attention-deficit/hyperactivity disorder. Pediatrics 2000;105:1158–70.
77. Palmer NB, Myers KM, Vander Stoep A, et al. Attention-deficit/hyperactivity disorder and telemental health. Curr Psychiatry Rep 2010;12(5):409–17.
78. Grady B, Myers KM, Nelson EL, et al. Evidence-based practice for telemental health. Telemed J E Health 2011;17:131–48.
79. Nelson EL, Davis K, Velasquez S. Ethical considerations in providing mental health services over videoconferencing. In: Myers K, Turvey C, editors.

Telemental health: clinical, technical and administrative foundations for evidence-based practice. New York: Elsevier; 2012. p. 47–60.

80. American Psychological Association (APA). Guidelines for the practice of telepsychology. 2013. Available at: http://www.apa.org/practice/guidelines/telepsychology.aspx. Accessed May 1, 2016.

81. Nelson E, Myers K. Child telemental health guidelines. American Telemedicine Association; in press.

82. Ohio Psychological Association. Ohio Psychological Association: areas of competence for psychologists in telepsychology. Columbus (OH): Ohio Psychological Association; 2012. Available at: http://www.ohpsych.org/about/files/2012/03/FINAL_COMPETENCY_DRAFT.pdf. Accessed May 1, 2016.

83. Goldstein F, Glueck D. Developing rapport and therapeutic alliance during telemental health sessions with children and adolescents. J Child Adolesc Psychopharmacol 2016;26(3):204–11.

84. American Telemedicine Association (ATA) Telepresenting Standards and Guidelines Working Group: expert consensus recommendations for videoconferencing-based telepresenting. 2013. Available at: http://www.americantelemed.org/resources/standards/ata-standards-guidelines/recommendations-for-videoconferencing-based-telepresenting#.U-rVffldWSo. Accessed May 1, 2016.

85. Jellinck M, Patel B, Froehle M, editors. Bright futures in practice: mental health—volume II. Tool kit. Arlington (VA): National Center for Education in Maternal and Child Health; 2002.

86. Swanson JM, Kraemer HC, Hinshaw SP, et al. Clinical relevance of the primary findings of the MTA: Success rates based on severity of ADHD and ODD symptoms at the end of treatment. J Am Acad Child Adolesc Psychiatry 2001;40:168–79.

87. Cain S, Sharp S. Telepharmacotherapy for children and adolescents. J Child Adolesc Psychopharmacol 2016;26(3):221–8.

88. Pelham WE Jr, Fabiano GA. Evidence-based psychosocial treatments for attention-deficit/hyperactivity disorder. J Clin Child Adolesc Psychol 2008;37:184–214.

89. Forehand R, Long N. Parenting the strong-willed child. 3rd edition. New York: McGraw-Hill; 2010.

90. Nelson E, Bui T, Sharp S. Telemental health competencies: training examples from a youth depression telemedicine clinic. In: Gregerson M, editor. Technology innovations for behavioral education. New York: Springer; 2011. p. 41–8.

91. Luxton DD, O'Brien K, McCann RA, et al. Home-based telemental healthcare safety planning: what you need to know. Telemed J E Health 2012;18:629–33.

92. US Department of Health and Human Services. The Affordable Care Act. 2010. Available at: http://www.hhs.gov/healthcare/about-the-law/read-the-law/index.html. Accessed May 1, 2015.

93. Fortney JC, Pyne JM, Edlund MJ, et al. A randomized trial of telemedicine-based collaborative care for depression. J Gen Intern Med 2007;22(8):1086–93.

94. Fortney JC, Pyne JM, Mouden SB, et al. Practice-based versus telemedicine-based collaborative care for depression in rural federally qualified health centers: a pragmatic randomized comparative effectiveness trial. Am J Psychiatry 2013;170(4):414–25.

95. McWilliams JK. Integrating telemental healthcare with the patient-centered medical home model. J Child Adolesc Psychopharmacol 2016;26(3):278–82.

96. Arora S, Thornton K, Komaromy M, et al. Demonopolizing medical knowledge. Acad Med 2014;89:30–2.

Developmental Surveillance and Screening in the Electronic Health Record

CrossMark

Timothy Ryan Smith, MD

KEYWORDS

- Electronic health record • Privacy • Developmental delay • Interoperability
- Clinical decision support • Health Information Exchange

KEY POINTS

- Define electronic health record (EHR) tools such as clinical decision support systems, registries, patient portals, and their application to developmental surveillance and screening.
- Discuss principles of interoperability and privacy and the challenges and opportunities posed for integration of developmental screening and surveillance into the EHR.
- Describe a conceptual framework that includes appropriate EHR tools in the completion of developmental screening and surveillance and referral to appropriate providers.

INTRODUCTION

Despite consensus among pediatricians about the importance of monitoring development in primary care, effective developmental screening and subsequent intervention remains challenging.[1] Developmental delay affects greater than 10% of pediatric patients[2] and nearly 50% of children fail to receive appropriate screening despite relative inexpensive cost and low difficulty.[3] Developmental delays require a medical evaluation that may include chromosomal analysis, MRI, and laboratory studies, as well as subspecialty medical and allied health evaluation.[4]

The electronic health record (EHR) provides an opportunity for prompt, consistent developmental assessment with clear, actionable protocols for intervention and follow-up, as well as tracking, to ensure practice improvement. Providers recognize the growing impact of EHR, positive and negative, on clinical care[5] and professional organizations attempt to support their members in creating efficient and efficacious systems. For example, the American Academy of Pediatrics (AAP) identifies the importance of health information technology in clinical care by setting the following priorities: (1) appropriate management and tracking of health data and services, (2)

Disclosure: None.
Department of Pediatrics, University of Kansas Medical Center, 3901 Rainbow Boulevard, MS 4004, Kansas City, KS 66160, USA
E-mail address: tsmith@kumc.edu

Pediatr Clin N Am 63 (2016) 933–943
http://dx.doi.org/10.1016/j.pcl.2016.06.014   pediatric.theclinics.com
0031-3955/16/$ – see front matter © 2016 Elsevier Inc. All rights reserved.

effective transfer of health information in patient care transitions, and (3) review of clinical data in continuous quality improvement.[6]

This article begins by defining developmental screening and surveillance. The next section introduces and applies the principles of interoperability and privacy to such evaluation in the EHR. Following, the current and future applications of tools, such as clinical decision support, registries, patient portals, and mobile technology is discussed. A conceptual framework summarizes the application of EHR tools. The conclusion reviews obstacles to implementation and future prospects. A glossary at the end of the article defines key terms and concepts from clinical informatics. Published literature on EHR and developmental screening and surveillance is limited, but representative articles are listed in **Box 1**.

DEVELOPMENTAL SURVEILLANCE AND SCREENING

Developmental surveillance addresses parental concerns and uses knowledgeable observation by a skilled practitioner to identify developmental problems.[7] The AAP states that appropriate developmental surveillance represents a "flexible, longitudinal, continuous, and cumulative process."[6,7] Bright Futures and AAP recommend developmental surveillance at all routine child health visits, also called well-child visits.[7]

In contrast, developmental screening involves use of a validated, standardized tool to identify and characterize risk.[1] The Council on Children with Disabilities identifies 20 developmental screening tools with appropriate validation, although this list is not exhaustive. Selection of an appropriate screening tool is challenging and often involves consideration of the following: the scope of developmental domains (grossmotor, fine-motor, social, language, and problem-solving) to be screened, scoring, other administrative needs, qualification for reimbursement by payers, and cost of tools.[1]

INTEROPERABILITY

Developmental issues require multidisciplinary collaboration and hinges on record systems sharing appropriate information. Interoperability, the ability of 2 or more systems to exchange and use information, is regularly discussed yet remains elusive in

---

Box 1
Literature on electronic health record tools and concepts and developmental screening and surveillance

Clinical Decision Support System (CDSS) - Carroll AE, Bauer NS, Dugan TM, et al. Use of a computerized decision aid for developmental surveillance and screening: a randomized clinical trial. JAMA Pediatr 2014;168(9):815–21.

CDSS - Council on Children With Disabilities, Section on Developmental Behavioral Pediatrics, Bright Futures Steering Committee, et al. Identifying infants and young children with developmental disorders in the medical home: an algorithm for developmental surveillance and screening. Pediatrics 2006;118(1):405–20.

Policy Statement or Multiple Tools - Council on Clinical Information Technology. Health information technology and the medical home. Pediatrics 2011;127(5):978–82.

Dashboards or CDSS - Jensen RE, Chan KS, Weiner JP, et al. Implementing electronic health record-based quality measures for developmental screening. Pediatrics 2009;124(4):e648–54.

EHR systems.[8] To achieve interoperability, common terminology must be determined, data must be efficiently collected, and information must be shared between institutions.

Common language is crucial to communication between independent systems. Data standards allow organizations to share information. Standardized screening tools and consistent coding allows sharing of pooled data and ensures consistent documentation across institutions. Systemized Nomenclature of Medicine clinical terms (SNOMED-CT) represents a national effort to create consistent terminology in medical records.[8] Pertinent data include diagnoses, screening outcomes, and interventions. Although screening tools may differ between institutions, common measures should be prioritized. Coding for a diagnosis and annotation for developmental delay or failed developmental screens in the problem list are appropriate targets.

Many challenges exist for tracking interventions for developmental screening and surveillance in primary care, but additional complexity emerges in linking medical specialists and other health providers, such as occupational and speech therapists, to pertinent information. Jensen and colleagues[9] evaluated developmental screening at 6 health care organizations and found that only one noted referral completion in the electronic medical record (EMR) and that institution did not capture this information in discrete data.

In addition, privacy and technical limitations have limited information exchange. Release of health information is guided by opt-in versus opt-out consent policies. Traditionally, the Health Information Portability and Accountability Act (HIPAA) has directed most practices to opt-in policies that require expressed permission to release pertinent health records,[10] whereas developments in the EHR, such as summary of care, have moved some institutions to use opt-out policies that allow more robust communication between primary care and specialty providers. With direction by professional organizations such as AAP and American Academy of Family Physicians, standard care summaries for developmental delays should be created and shared across different EHR vendor platforms.

These transition documents are important to meaningful use and the patient-centered medical home. Furthermore, these resources are moving toward push, rather than pull, modalities. For pull requests, an outside system specifically requests information, whereas push information is sent automatically from one facility to another. Pushing pertinent information to specialty providers from referring or primary care providers and vice versa improves communication critical to patient care.

Tools exist to connect data sets, although these tools are limited between distinct institutions and EHR vendors. Korzeniewski and colleagues[11] used Centers for Disease Control and Prevention (CDC) software to merge 2 institutional data sets to identify children who failed to receive a newborn screen and examine the reasons for failure. One can imagine the benefit of shared information between health and educational institutions on development. Health providers could provide schools with medical diagnoses and screenings and anticipated educational deficits. At the same time, schools could communicate in place of describe provided services, such as speech, physical, and occupational therapy, as well as progress and pitfalls in attainment. Bidirectional communication using EHRs, health information exchanges (HIEs), and registries is critical to safe, efficient, and efficacious multidisciplinary care.

HIEs remain critical for patient-centered care across practice settings,[12] but their implementation has lagged behind other elements of meaningful use. Exchanges have grown at the local, state, regional, and national levels with public and private funding since passage of the Health Information Technology for Economic and Clinical Health (HITECH) Act in 2009.[8] Barriers for successful implementation of HIE are broad but can be categorized into incomplete information, access to exchanges, and organization of data.[13]

THE HEALTH INFORMATION PORTABILITY AND ACCOUNTABILITY ACT

Most providers have been exposed to data security protections via HIPAA. This legislation formalized information security in medical records and is guided by the 3 core principles of information security: confidentiality, availability, and integrity.[8] Familiar to patients and providers, confidentiality prevents data loss and inappropriate sharing with organizations or individuals. EHR systems have improved availability of medical records to patients and providers, although numerous contingencies, including weather, network failures, and hardware issues, must be considered. Patient portals have provided greater access to personal health records via the patient's home computer or smartphone. Ensuring that families have access to their own health data is countered by the need to contextualize this information with appropriate resources from reliable sources such as the CDC and AAP. Data integrity ensures that health information is protected against modification from unauthorized entities and protected against loss or corruption. Regional and national registries for developmental data could complement institutional efforts in data back-up and best practices. Consequences for cognitive functioning, functional abilities, and medical or social needs make security for developmental data particularly important. Indeed, data security remains a persistent issue with greater than 1.8 million medical-related breaches in 2013 in the United States.[8]

CLINICAL DECISION SUPPORT SYSTEMS

Hoyt and Yoshihashi[8] describe clinical decision support systems (CDSS) as "any software designed to directly aid in clinical decision making in which characteristics of individual patients are matched to a computerized knowledge base for the purpose of generating patient specific assessments or recommendations." CDSS uses systems within the EMR to direct appropriate practice and has been proven to increase adherence to evidence-based care and decrease medication and practice errors.[14] Clinical resources such as iConsult and clinical practice guidelines from AAP can guide design of tools such as graphs, flowsheets, order sets, patient reminders, and EHR alerts.

Applied to developmental screening and surveillance, CDSS could flag children with failed developmental screens and recommend medical or ancillary health intervention or evaluation, ensure that each routine care visit has appropriate screening or surveillance reviewed by provider and other health care staff, or consolidate fragments of pertinent information on development to a single location. Carroll and colleagues[15] used computerized CDSSs and improved rates of developmental screening at 4 clinics. Implementation of clinical decision support should involve all strata of the health care system from individual practice to national and international health organizations.

DASHBOARDS

Dashboards may guide appropriate clinical screening and interventions by presenting pooled data to providers and administrators in a central location.[16,17] Partnering with accountable care organizations and other insurance entities, institutions could configure EHRs to analyze and organize claims data for developmental screening in dashboards. Such efforts depend on consistent documentation, reliable claims data transferred into the EHR, and provider engagement.[18] Studies suggest that well-designed dashboards move physicians to more consistent practices, although much greater examination is needed.[19,20]

PATIENT PORTALS

Patient portals and patient-input questionnaires may dramatically change clinical care in the future. Patients may complete health screenings, including developmental milestones, before arrival at an appointment, allow providers to review such results, involve additional health providers, and plan further interventions in before-visit huddles. These forms could be completed at a clinic computer or tablet kiosks or, preferably, on a computer, tablet, smartphone, or other internet-enabled device at home. The success of these efforts, as well as many others surrounding health and education, depend on closing the digital divide.[21] Studies suggest that patients may prefer electronic questionnaires to paper ones.[22,23] Jensen and colleagues[9] recognized the potential gains in tracking developmental screening and associated interventions but also recognized potential obstacles.

Ultimately, initial screens could direct deeper investigation into potential delays in distinct domains of development such as language. Suggested delays in language could lead to more involved questions to further classify or confirm such a diagnosis. This nesting allows automation of more involved examination of flagged domains with limited staff resources and limited expertise in the primary care setting.[24] This new direction will likely require the creation of new tools and subsequent validation.

CONSUMER HEALTH INFORMATICS

Patient interest in health information has spurred consumer health informatics. Digital content has exercised greater influence on health decisions than traditional media such as print, television, and radio.[8] Online resources are quickly approaching the influence of physician advice in health decisions. Vaccine hesitancy provides an illustrative example. Parents cite the Internet as an influence for electing to defer or decline vaccinations due to concern for an increased risk for autism or other developmental delay with immunization.[25,26] Components of the Affordable Care Act incentivize accountable care organizations to engage patients in health actions such as wellness. Indeed, meaningful use heralds "engaging patients and families" and "empowering individuals."[8]

The burden for validating health resources has fallen on health care providers.[27] With greater than 40,000 health applications (apps) on iTunes, this task has been increasingly difficult. Healthy Children and ADHD Tracker represent mobile apps related to childhood development supported by the AAP for parents, yet represent a small fraction of the apps available.

MOBILE HEALTH

Smartphones, tablets, and wearable technologies promise to impact health, in general, and, developmental surveillance and screening, in particular, in similar ways to travel, finance, journalism, and navigation. Query of the apps for child development yields numerous results, but apps from dependable pediatric health sources, such as HealthyChildren, may be obscured by less reliable ones. With the emergence of consumer health informatics, providers are compelled to direct patients to the best apps, Web sites, and other resources.

REGISTRIES

Numerous risk factors confer increased or decreased risk for delays, including gestational age, medical comorbidities, maternal education, poor weight gain, family history, and abnormal past results for surveillance and screening. Numerous studies and registries[28,29] have highlighted increased risk for developmental delay, but literature that examines the utilization of patient risk factors to direct developmental screening and interventions is limited. A comprehensive national registry on developmental milestones and outcomes could complement current registries by documenting development in specific populations.[30–32] Management of data within registries remains challenging and, ultimately, should be structured to import data from various EHR systems and export data seamlessly when requested.

CLINICAL PRACTICE GUIDELINES

Numerous clinical practices guidelines by the AAP, American Academy of Neurology, and Child Neurology Society address the diagnosis and management of developmental delay. Elements of clinical practice guidelines are implemented in EHRs by action alerts, order sets, and clinical reports. Efforts have produced mixed results[8] but likely will improve as data becomes more standard, specific, and retrievable.

QUALITY IMPROVEMENT

In addition to improving longitudinal developmental progress for individual children, developmental screening and surveillance in the EMR promises to track and improve practices at provider, practice, state, and national levels.[15] Normative data could better validate tools and direct standard practices. For example, an EHR could compare the percentage of failed developmental screens and referral for medical and ancillary health evaluation, and build systems to better ensure that appropriate action is taken for failed developmental screens. Population-based data could classify risk and target interventions and outreach programs.

OBSTACLES TO USE

Proprietary content complicates integration of developmental screening. Some established developmental screening tools, such as the Ages and Stages Questionnaire (ASQ) and Parents Evaluation of Developmental Status (PEDS) have restrictions on placing items into EHRs with operating their own Web portal for inputting data.[33,34] Some developmental screens, such as Survey of Well-Being for Children (SWYC), were created without intellectual property restrictions but have more limited literature on validity.[35,36]

Many providers complain that medical practice exists in silos with practitioners at one facility often unaware of completed or pending interventions at another facility. Many early interventions programs are managed by state agencies outside traditional health recordkeeping systems, making communication between primary care and referral providers through the EHR difficult. Connecting to institutions outside of conventional health systems is instrumental for comprehensive care of children with developmental delays. An AAP policy statement emphasizes this by highlighting the role of multidisciplinary health professionals, including early childhood educators, child psychologists, audiologists, social workers, physical therapists, and occupational therapists, in the evaluation and treatment of developmental disorders.[1]

Non-English language patients provide a challenge to adoption of EHR systems as well as specific tools.[37] Tools such as the patient portal may afford parents and their children access to their health records and improved communication providers and other health care staff but non-English language poses a significant barrier.[21]

In addition to difficulty with the EHR, non-English language may present an independent risk factor for delayed or missed developmental delays. Indeed, validated translations of developmental screening tools have lagged behind growing language diversity of patients in pediatric practice.[38]

CONCEPTUAL FRAMEWORK

All well-child visits should include developmental surveillance or screening. **Fig. 1** presents a conceptual framework for implementing EHR tools for developmental screening. Visits outside of the 9, 18, and 30 months visits without previous or new developmental concerns should complete surveillance. Parents could be better prepared for developmental discussions by providing pertinent, reliable resources in advance. In addition, pushing developmental questionnaires via a patient portal accessed via a home computer, tablet, or mobile phone preceding a visit could provide parents more time for attention to developmental concerns. Clinical decision support could flag failed milestones that merit screening or intervention for providers.

Appropriate developmental screening and surveillance tools should have seamless integration into EHRs. Screening tools must boast adequate validation in published literature (see Box 1 in **Fig. 1**). Such screens should be used on all children at the 9, 18, and 30 month visits and all children with parental or provider concerns for other visits (see Box 2 in **Fig. 1**). Clinical decision support could alert providers to patients that may benefit from early intervention or medical evaluation (see Box 2 in **Fig. 1**). Physician dashboards could direct appropriate referral practices by reporting referrals against the number of flagged developmental screens compared with established benchmarks (see Box 3 in **Fig. 1**).

Secure, relevant HIPAA-compliant data are transmitted to medical subspecialists and allied health professionals via HIEs or registries (see Box 3 in **Fig. 1**). Diagnosis and management should be returned to the primary care provider through exchanges or registries (see Box 3 in **Fig. 1**).

The wealth of information gleaned from primary care providers, medical subspecialists, and allied health professionals via registries could further validate screening tools and target interventions for individuals and populations (see Box 4 in **Fig. 1**).

SUMMARY

Often, developmental screening and surveillance produces a binary result at a particular point in time. A child either does or does not meet a milestone at one visit. Comparison to past results may not be easily available and requires laborious chart review between encounters. Annotation of failed screening in the problem list draws attention to these issues in future visits. However, such efforts may inconsistently draw attention to the issue.[39] Sheldrick[24] proposed a "developmental growth curve" to graphically follow developmental milestones over time. Growth curves for weight, height, and body mass index allows providers to identify and address growth trends before they reach abnormal values such as the 5% percentile. Graphically identifying developmental lags may provide valuable information for diagnosis and prognosis of developmental conditions.

Jensen and colleagues[9] described 3 targets for improvements of developmental screening through EHRs: administration of appropriate tool, identification of abnormal results, and follow-up for indicated patients and subsequent primary care provider engagement. EHRs have presented providers with a greater burden for

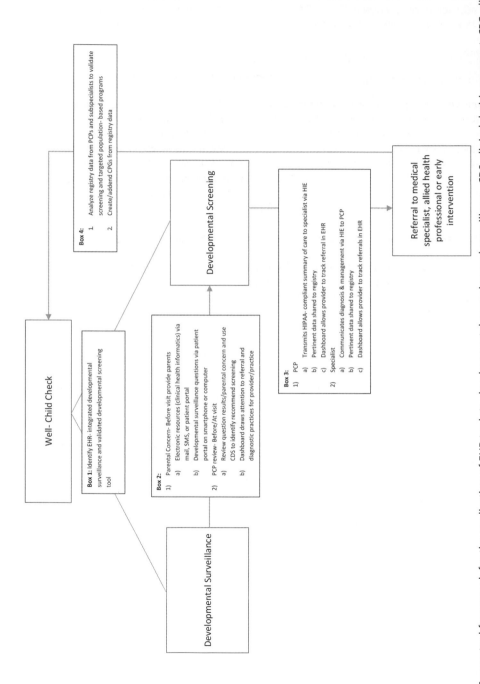

Fig. 1. Conceptual framework for the application of EHR tools to developmental screening and surveillance. CDS, clinical decision support; CPG, clinical practice guideline; PCP, primary care provider; SMS, short message service.

documentation; however, collaboration between providers, health systems, and governmental and professional organizations promises meeting these objectives and improving clinical care. Informaticists, health care providers, legislators, and administrators should advocate for integrated solutions.

Glossary
  Data integration: Combining data from multiple sources into a single view.
  Discrete or structured data: Information that is limited to numerical values or pre-specified categories.
  Electronic medical record (EMR) and electronic health record (EHR): The EMR represents the sum of data in the clinical setting, whereas the EHR more broadly describes the sum of data across the entire continuum of care.
  Health information exchange (HIE): Electronic movement of health-related information among organizations according to nationally recognized standards.
  Health Information Technology for Economic and Clinical Health (HITECH) Act: 2009 federal legislation that provided incentives through Medicaid and Medicare reimbursement for the adoption and advanced use of EHRs. Meaningful use was an important component of HITECH.
  Interoperability: Ability for independent systems and devices to exchange and interpret shared data.
  Meaningful use: Established by HITECH Act, MU created 3 stages for process measures for implementing appropriate functionality in EHR.

Adapted from Haas[40] and Hoyt[8]

REFERENCES

1. Council on Children With Disabilities, Section on Developmental Behavioral Pediatrics, Bright Futures Steering Committee, et al. Identifying infants and young children with developmental disorders in the medical home: an algorithm for developmental surveillance and screening. Pediatrics 2006;118(1):405–20.
2. Boyle CA, Decouflé P, Yeargin-Allsopp M. Prevalence and health impact of developmental disabilities in US children. Pediatrics 1994;93(3):399–403.
3. Sices L, Decouflé P, Yeargin-Allsopp M. How do primary care physicians identify young children with developmental delays? A national survey. J Dev Behav Pediatr 2003;24(6):409–17.
4. Shevell M, Ashwal S, Donley D, et al. Practice parameter: evaluation of the child with global developmental delay: report of the Quality Standards Subcommittee of the American Academy of Neurology and The Practice Committee of the Child Neurology Society. Neurology 2003;60(3):367–80.
5. Lau F, Price M, Boyd J, et al. Impact of electronic medical record on physician practice in office settings: a systematic review. BMC Med Inform Decis Mak 2012;12:10.
6. Council on Clinical Information Technology. Health information technology and the medical home. Pediatrics 2011;127(5):978–82.
7. Developmental surveillance and screening of infants and young children. Pediatrics 2001;108(1):192–6.
8. Hoyt R, Yoshihashi AK. Health informatics: practical guide for healthcare and information technology professionals. 2014.
9. Jensen RE, Chan KS, Weiner JP, et al. Implementing electronic health record-based quality measures for developmental screening. Pediatrics 2009;124(4): e648–54.

10. Littenberg B, MacLean CD. Passive consent for clinical research in the age of HI-PAA. J Gen Intern Med 2006;21(3):207–11.
11. Korzeniewski SJ, Grigorescu V, Copeland G, et al. Methodological innovations in data gathering: newborn screening linkage with live births records, Michigan, 1/2007-3/2008. Matern Child Health J 2010;14(3):360–4.
12. Richardson JE, Vest JR, Green CM, et al. A needs assessment of health information technology for improving care coordination in three leading patient-centered medical homes. J Am Med Inform Assoc 2015;22(4):815–20.
13. Eden KB, Totten AM, Kassakian SZ, et al. Barriers and facilitators to exchanging health information: a systematic review. Int J Med Inform 2016;88:44–51.
14. Wajngurt D, Hong F, Chaudhry R, et al. EpiPortal: an electronic decision support system for infection control. AMIA Annu Symp Proc 2006;1132.
15. Carroll AE, Bauer NS, Dugan TM, et al. Use of a computerized decision aid for developmental surveillance and screening: a randomized clinical trial. JAMA Pediatr 2014;168(9):815–21.
16. Koopman RJ, Kochendorfer KM, Moore JL, et al. A diabetes dashboard and physician efficiency and accuracy in accessing data needed for high-quality diabetes care. Ann Fam Med 2011;9(5):398–405.
17. Linder JA, Schnipper JL, Tsurikova R, et al. Electronic health record feedback to improve antibiotic prescribing for acute respiratory infections. Am J Manag Care 2010;16(12 Suppl HIT):e311–9.
18. Berkowitz SA, Ishii L, Schulz J, et al. Academic Medical Centers Forming Accountable Care Organizations and Partnering With Community Providers: the experience of the Johns Hopkins Medicine alliance for patients. Acad Med 2016;91(3):328–32.
19. Hartzler AL, Chaudhuri S, Fey BC, et al. Integrating patient-reported outcomes into spine surgical care through visual dashboards: lessons learned from human-centered design. EGEMS (Wash DC) 2015;3(2):1133.
20. Redwood S, Ngwenya NB, Hodson J, et al. Effects of a computerized feedback intervention on safety performance by junior doctors: results from a randomized mixed method study. BMC Med Inform Decis Mak 2013;13:63.
21. Sarkar U, Karter AJ, Liu JY, et al. Social disparities in internet patient portal use in diabetes: evidence that the digital divide extends beyond access. J Am Med Inform Assoc 2011;18(3):318–21.
22. Pouwer F, Snoek FJ, van der Ploeg HM, et al. A comparison of the standard and the computerized versions of the Well-being Questionnaire (WBQ) and the Diabetes Treatment Satisfaction Questionnaire (DTSQ). Qual Life Res 1998;7(1):33–8.
23. Caro JJ Sr, Caro I, Caro J, et al. Does electronic implementation of questionnaires used in asthma alter responses compared with paper implementation? Qual Life Res 2001;10(8):683–91.
24. Sheldrick RC, Perrin EC. Surveillance of children's behavior and development: practical solutions for primary care. J Dev Behav Pediatr 2009;30(2):151–3.
25. Stahl JP, Cohen R, Denis F, et al. The impact of the web and social networks on vaccination. New challenges and opportunities offered to fight against vaccine hesitancy. Med Mal Infect 2016;46(3):117–22.
26. Shoup JA, Wagner NM, Kraus CR, et al. Development of an interactive social media tool for parents with concerns about vaccines. Health Educ Behav 2015;42(3):302–12.
27. Eysenbach G. Medicine 2.0: social networking, collaboration, participation, apomediation, and openness. J Med Internet Res 2008;10(3):e22.

28. Woolfenden S, Eapen V, Axelsson E, et al. Who is our cohort: recruitment, representativeness, baseline risk and retention in the "Watch Me Grow" study? BMC Pediatr 2016;16(1):46.
29. Schlapbach LJ, Adams M, Proietti E, et al. Outcome at two years of age in a Swiss national cohort of extremely preterm infants born between 2000 and 2008. BMC Pediatr 2012;12:198.
30. Stoll BJ, Hansen NI, Bell EF, et al. Trends in care practices, morbidity, and mortality of extremely preterm neonates, 1993-2012. JAMA 2015;314(10):1039–51.
31. Roberts AE, Nixon C, Steward CG, et al. The Barth Syndrome Registry: distinguishing disease characteristics and growth data from a longitudinal study. Am J Med Genet A 2012;158A(11):2726–32.
32. Brandlistuen RE, Stene-Larsen K, Holmstrøm H, et al. Occurrence and predictors of developmental impairments in 3-year-old children with congenital heart defects. J Dev Behav Pediatr 2011;32(7):526–32.
33. Available at: http://agesandstages.com/products-services/asq-online/. Accessed April 27, 2016.
34. Available at: http://www.pedstest.com/default.aspx. Accessed April 27, 2016.
35. Sheldrick RC, Perrin EC. Evidence-based milestones for surveillance of cognitive, language, and motor development. Acad Pediatr 2013;13(6):577–86.
36. Whitesell NR, Sarche M, Trucksess C, et al. The survey of well-being of young children: results of a feasibility study with American Indian and Alaska Native Communities. Infant Ment Health J 2015;36(5):483–505.
37. Li C, West-Strum D. Patient panel of underserved populations and adoption of electronic medical record systems by office-based physicians. Health Serv Res 2010;45(4):963–84.
38. El-Behadli AF, Neger EN, Perrin EC, et al. Translations of developmental screening instruments: an evidence map of available research. J Dev Behav Pediatr 2015;36(6):471–83.
39. Mowery DL, Jordan P, Wiebe J, et al. Semantic annotation of clinical events for generating a problem list. AMIA Annu Symp Proc 2013;2013:1032–41.
40. Haas JP. Glossary of terms for information technology and pearls of wisdom for implementation and use. Am J Infect Control 2015;43(6):551–3.

Index

Note: Page numbers of article titles are in **boldface** type.

Pediatr Clin N Am 63 (2016) 945–954
http://dx.doi.org/10.1016/S0031-3955(16)41071-0
0031-3955/16/$ – see front matter

pediatric.theclinics.com

UNITED STATES POSTAL SERVICE® Statement of Ownership, Management, and Circulation (All Periodicals Publications Except Requester Publications)

1. Publication Title	2. Publication Number		3. Filing Date
PEDIATRIC CLINICS OF NORTH AMERICA	424 – 66		9/18/2016

4. Issue Frequency	5. Number of Issues Published Annually	3. Annual Subscription Price
FEB, APR, JUN, AUG, OCT, DEC	6	$200.00

7. Complete Mailing Address of Known Office of Publication (Not printer) (Street, city, county, state, and ZIP+4®)

ELSEVIER INC.
360 PARK AVENUE SOUTH
NEW YORK, NY 10010-1710

Contact Person
STEPHEN R. BUSHING

Telephone (Include area code)
215-239-3688

8. Complete Mailing Address of Headquarters or General Business Office of Publisher (Not printer)

ELSEVIER INC.
360 PARK AVENUE SOUTH
NEW YORK, NY 10010-1710

9. Full Names and Complete Mailing Addresses of Publisher, Editor, and Managing Editor (Do not leave blank)

Publisher (Name and complete mailing address)

LINDA BELFUS, ELSEVIER INC.
1600 JOHN F KENNEDY BLVD. SUITE 1800
PHILADELPHIA, PA 19103-2899

Editor (Name and complete mailing address)

KERRY HOLLAND, ELSEVIER INC.
1600 JOHN F KENNEDY BLVD. SUITE 1800
PHILADELPHIA, PA 19103-2899

Managing Editor (Name and complete mailing address)

ADRIANNE BRIGIDO, ELSEVIER INC.
1600 JOHN F KENNEDY BLVD. SUITE 1800
PHILADELPHIA, PA 19103-2899

10. Owner (Do not leave blank. If the publication is owned by a corporation, give the name and address of the corporation immediately followed by the names and addresses of all stockholders owning or holding 1 percent or more of the total amount of stock. If not owned by a corporation, give the names and addresses of the individual owners. If owned by a partnership or other unincorporated firm, give its name and address as well as those of each individual owner. If the publication is published by a nonprofit organization, give its name and address.)

Full Name	Complete Mailing Address
WHOLLY OWNED SUBSIDIARY OF REED/ELSEVIER, US HOLDINGS	1600 JOHN F KENNEDY BLVD. SUITE 1800 PHILADELPHIA, PA 19103-2899

11. Known Bondholders, Mortgagees, and Other Security Holders Owning or Holding 1 Percent or More of Total Amount of Bonds, Mortgages, or Other Securities. If none, check box → ☐ None

Full Name	Complete Mailing Address
N/A	

12. Tax Status (For completion by nonprofit organizations authorized to mail at nonprofit rates) (Check one)
The purpose, function, and nonprofit status of this organization and the exempt status for federal income tax purposes:
☐ Has Not Changed During Preceding 12 Months
☐ Has Changed During Preceding 12 Months (Publisher must submit explanation of change with this statement)

13. Publication Title	14. Issue Date for Circulation Data Below
PEDIATRIC CLINICS OF NORTH AMERICA	JUNE 2016

15. Extent and Nature of Circulation			Average No. Copies Each Issue During Preceding 12 Months	No. Copies of Single Issue Published Nearest to Filing Date
a. Total Number of Copies (Net press run)			1091	1148
b. Paid Circulation (By Mail and Outside the Mail)	(1)	Mailed Outside-County Paid Subscriptions Stated on PS Form 3541 (Include paid distribution above nominal rate, advertiser's proof copies, and exchange copies)	423	557
	(2)	Mailed In-County Paid Subscriptions Stated on PS Form 3541 (Include paid distribution above nominal rate, advertiser's proof copies, and exchange copies)	0	0
	(3)	Paid Distribution Outside the Mails Including Sales Through Dealers and Carriers, Street Vendors, Counter Sales, and Other Paid Distribution Outside USPS®	307	397
	(4)	Paid Distribution by Other Classes of Mail Through the USPS (e.g. First-Class Mail®)	0	0
c. Total Paid Distribution [Sum of 15b (1), (2), (3), and (4)]			730	954
d. Free or Nominal Rate Distribution (By Mail and Outside the Mail)	(1)	Free or Nominal Rate Outside-County Copies included on PS Form 3541	46	109
	(2)	Free or Nominal Rate In-County Copies Included on PS Form 3541	0	0
	(3)	Free or Nominal Rate Copies Mailed at Other Classes Through the USPS (e.g. First-Class Mail)	0	0
	(4)	Free or Nominal Rate Distribution Outside the Mail (Carriers or other means)	0	0
e. Total Free or Nominal Rate Distribution (Sum of 15d (1), (2), (3) and (4))			46	109
f. Total Distribution (Sum of 15c and 15e)			776	1063
g. Copies not Distributed (See Instructions to Publishers #4 (page #3))			315	85
h. Total (Sum of 15f and g)			1091	1148
i. Percent Paid (15c divided by 15f times 100)			94%	90%

If you are claiming electronic copies, go to line 16 on page 3. If you are not claiming electronic copies, skip to line 17 on page 3.

16. Electronic Copy Circulation	Average No. Copies Each Issue During Preceding 12 Months	No. Copies of Single Issue Published Nearest to Filing Date
a. Paid Electronic Copies ▶	0	0
b. Total Paid Print Copies (Line 15c) + Paid Electronic Copies (Line 16a) ▶	760	954
c. Total Print Distribution (Line 15f) + Paid Electronic Copies (Line 16a) ▶	776	1063
d. Percent Paid (Both Print & Electronic Copies) (16b divided by 16c × 100) ▶	94%	90%

☒ I certify that 50% of all my distributed copies (electronic and print) are paid above a nominal price.

17. Publication of Statement of Ownership
☒ If the publication is a general publication, publication of this statement is required. Will be printed in the OCTOBER 2016 issue of this publication.
☐ Publication not required.

18. Signature and Title of Editor, Publisher, Business Manager, or Owner

Stephen R. Bushing — Date 9/18/2016

STEPHEN F. BUSHING - INVENTORY DISTRIBUTION CONTROL MANAGER

I certify that all information furnished on this form is true and complete. I understand that anyone who furnishes false or misleading information on this form or who omits material or information requested on the form may be subject to criminal sanctions (including fines and imprisonment) and/or civil sanctions (including civil penalties).

PS Form 3526, July 2014 (Page 3 of 4) PSN 7530-01-000-9931 PRIVACY NOTICE: See our privacy policy on www.usps.com.

PS Form 3526, July 2014 (Page 1 of 4 (see instructions page 4)) PSN 7530-01-000-9931 PRIVACY NOTICE: See our privacy policy on www.usps.com.

CONTINUING MEDICAL EDUCATION SUPPLEMENT

PEDIATRIC CLINICS OF NORTH AMERICA

Sponsored by
Elsevier Office of Continuing Medical Education

Based on the issue
Childhood Development and Behavior (Vol 63:5), October 2016

Test expires 12 months following publication date.

Test Publication Date: October 2016   Test expires: October 31, 2017*

*You must have a current subscription in order to claim credit. Please complete the test before your CME subscription expires.

TEST NO. PCL63:5 • OCTOBER, 2016

W. B. SAUNDERS COMPANY
An imprint of Elsevier, Inc.

Elsevier Inc.
1600 John F. Kennedy Blvd., Suite 1800
Philadelphia, PA 19103-2899

http://www.us.elsevierhealth.com

CONTINUING MEDICAL EDUCATION
SUPPLEMENT TO PEDIATRIC CLINICS OF NORTH AMERICA
ISSN 1557-8135   **OCTOBER 2016**

CHANGE OF ADDRESS
We cannot score tests submitted after the 12-month deadline has expired. Please notify us immediately of any change in address to ensure that your test booklet reaches you in a timely manner. Send address changes, along with a copy of the mailing label from your test booklet, to:

Elsevier US Books Customer Services
3251 Riverport Lane
Maryland Heights, MO 63043, USA
(800) 654-2452 (Toll Free US and Canada)
(314) 453-7041 (Outside US and Canada)

Email: journalscustomerservice-usa@elsevier.com
URL: http://www.theclinics.com/

TEST NO. PCL63:5   •   OCTOBER, 2016

INSTRUCTIONS FOR COMPLETING THE EXAMINATION FOR CREDIT

The test booklet has been mailed to you for your convenience; however, all examinations must be taken online in order to receive credit.

Please register online at www.theclinics.com/home/cme using the account number provided on the mailing label of this test booklet. Instructions for completing the test are provided on the website. With the online service, readers will benefit from the convenience of instant scoring and credit.

Test questions will be available online for 12 months.

Technical support is available Monday through Friday during the hours of 7:30 am to 6:00 pm EST:

Elsevier US Books Customer Services
3251 Riverport Lane
Maryland Heights, MO 63043, USA
(800) 654-2452 (Toll Free US and Canada)
(314) 453-7041 (Outside US and Canada)

Email: journalscustomerservice-usa@elsevier.com
URL: http://www.theclinics.com/

If you do not have access to a computer, please call Customer Service to obtain an answer sheet. Please return your answer sheet via mail; *faxed answer sheets will not be accepted.* Remember to complete both the test and the subsequent program evaluation. Please allow 6 to 8 weeks for processing and scoring answer sheets submitted in this manner.

TEST NO. PCL63:5 • OCTOBER, 2016

Impact of Military Deployment on the Development and Behavior of Children

1. According to this article, which of the following is TRUE?

   A. the After Deployment, Adaptive Parenting Tools (ADAPT) is a parenting support intervention for National Guard and Reserve families

   B. Families Overcoming Under Stress (FOCUS) is an online support program for active military duty families

   C. four stages of the deployment cycle have been identified: Predeployment, Deployment, Sustainment and Postdeployment

   D. military personnel are less likely to be married with children compared to their civilian counterparts

Growing Up – or Not – with Gun Violence

2. Programs have been developed to educate children on gun violence and safety. Which of the following statements regarding gun violence and safety education for children is TRUE?

   A. the Center to Prevent Handgun Violence program, "Straight Talk About Risks," is the only program proven to prevent children from handling guns

   B. the Center to Prevent Handgun Violence program, "Straight Talk About Risks," targets high school students

   C. the National Rifle Association's Eddie Eagle GunSafe Program is designed for teenage students

   D. through research, the National Rifle Association's Eddie Eagle GunSafe Program has not been proven to be effective

TEST NO. PCL63:5 • OCTOBER, 2016

775 **Development in Children of Immigrant Families**

3. Which of the following are two of the three fundamental developmental processes for the immigrant child?

   A. bilingualism and marginalization
   B. ethnic identity formation and acculturation
   C. ethnic identity formation and migration context
   D. marginalization and migration context

827 **Increased Screen Time, Implications for Early Childhood Development and Behavior**

4. Creative problem solving, attention span and tolerance of brain downtime are examples of:

   A. cognitive areas of development which are positively affected by digital product use
   B. cognitive areas of development which may be negatively affected by digital product use
   C. socio-emotional areas of development which are positively affected by digital product use
   D. socio-emotional areas of development which may be negatively affected by digital product use

851 **Whittling Down the Wait Time**

5. Which of the following statements regarding the Autism Diagnostic Observation Schedule (ADOS) is TRUE?

   A. the ADOS diagnostic tool must be performed in order to assign a diagnosis of autism spectrum disorder
   B. the ADOS has become the gold standard diagnostic tool for autism spectrum disorder diagnosis T
   C. the ADOS is a play-based standardized assessment for children under 12 months
   D. the ADOS must be performed by a specially trained psychiatrist

86\ **Early Identification and Treatment of Antisocial Behavior**

6. Callous-unemotional traits are characterized by all of the following EXCEPT:

   A. intense display of reactive emotion
   B. lack of empathy T
   C. lack of guilt T
   D. restricted display of affect

87\ **Social Media: Challenges and Concerns for Families**

7. The Children's Online Privacy Protection Act (COPPA) has set the minimum age of use for social media sites as:

   A. 10
   B. 13
   C. 15
   D. 16

TEST NO. PCL63:5 • OCTOBER, 2016

88?

Transitions in Healthcare: What Can We Learn From Our Experience with Cystic Fibrosis

8. According to the article, which of the following statements regarding transition to adult care is TRUE?

   A. parental involvement in the transition to adult care is often counter-productive
   B. patient readiness to transition into adult care begins between ages 16–18
   C. transition to adult care can begin at age 13 or earlier
   D. transition to adult care can begin between ages 18 and 21

913

A Review of Pediatric Telemental Health

9. According to the article, approximately what percentage of children and adolescents in the United States have diagnosable psychiatric disorders?

   A. 20%
   B. 31%
   C. 35%
   D. 41%

873

Specialized Behavioral Therapies for Children with Special Needs

10. The goals of which of the following treatments focuses on reducing mental health issues in middle childhood by identifying negative thoughts, beliefs and perceptions, and replacing them with more constructive emotional responses, behavior and thinking?

    A. attachment and biobehavioral catch-up
    B. cognitive behavior therapy --
    C. dialectical behavior therapy
    D. Parent-Child Interaction Therapy

899

Integrating Pediatric Palliative Care into the School and Community

11. Which of the following statements regarding comprehensive pediatric palliative care (CPPC) is TRUE?

    A. while CPPC addresses the physical needs of children with chronic health conditions, opportunity to address the child's emotional and spiritual needs still exists
    B. CPPC is a philosophy of care for children facing a life-limiting condition who have a life expectancy of months
    C. CPPC has been widely and successfully integrated into schools across the United States thanks to education and civil rights legislation
    D. a major challenge to CPPC is out-of-hospital do-not-resuscitate orders

933 **Developmental Surveillance and Screening in the Electronic Health Record**

12. Which of the following is an obstacle to using the electronic health record for developmental screening and surveillance?

    A. Clinical Decision Support System
    B. communication between programs outside of conventional health systems and primary care providers
    C. health information exchanges
    D. the Systemized Nomenclature of Medicine clinical terms

EVALUATION FORM

Elsevier Office of Continuing Medical Education is committed to excellence in continuing education, and your opinions are critical to us in this effort. To assist us in evaluating the effectiveness of this activity and to make recommendations for future educational offerings, please take a few minutes to complete this evaluation form.

You must complete this evaluation form online to receive credit for this activity.

Please Rate this CME Activity

	Poor	Fair	Good	Very Good	Excellent
Overall Evaluation	1	2	(3)	4	5
Content	1	2	(3)	4	5
Usefulness	1	2	(3)	4	5
Quality	1	2	(3)	4	5

Please rate how well this activity met the educational objectives

Review the effects of factors such as military deployment, gun violence and increased screen time on children's developmental health.

Strongly Disagree	Disagree	Neutral	Agree	Strongly Agree
1	2	3	(4)	5

Discuss the identification and management of autism and antisocial behavior in children.

Strongly Disagree	Disagree	Neutral	Agree	Strongly Agree
1	2	3	(4)	5

TEST NO. PCL63:5 • OCTOBER, 2016

Recognize developments in pediatric telemental health, behavioral therapies and palliative care.

Strongly Disagree	Disagree	Neutral	Agree	Strongly Agree
1	2	3	(4)	5

Was presentation fair, balanced and free of commercial bias?

☑ Yes   ☐ No

If no, please explain:

Will the information presented encourage you to make any changes in your practice?   *yes*

If yes, please describe any change(s) you plan to make in your practice?
   More aware of challenges

If no, please indicate your reasons for making this decision:
   a. Information presented confirmed my current practice
   b. Information presented did not convince me of need to change
   c. Barriers prevent making a change

How many patients do you see per month?   *200*

What topics would you like to see in future CME activities?

Do you wish to be notified by email when new educational programs are offered by Elsevier Office of Continuing Medical Education?
   ☐   Yes   ☑   No

All evaluation responses are confidential.